ERADICATING DEAFNESS?

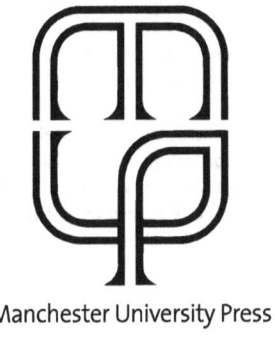

Manchester University Press

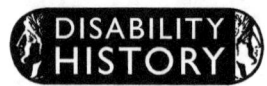

Series editors
Dr Julie Anderson, Professor Walton O. Schalick, III

This series published by Manchester University Press responds to the growing interest in disability as a discipline worthy of historical research. The series has a broad international historical remit, encompassing issues that include class, race, gender, age, war, medical treatment, professionalisation, environments, work, institutions and cultural and social aspects of disablement including representations of disabled people in literature, film, art and the media.

Already published

Deafness, community and culture in Britain: leisure and cohesion, 1945-1995
Martin Atherton

Disability in industrial Britain: A cultural and literary history of impairment in the coal industry, 1880–1948
Kirsti Bohata, Alexandra Jones, Mike Mantin and Steven Thompson

Disability and the Victorians: Attitudes, interventions, legacies
Iain Hutchinson

Rethinking modern prostheses in Anglo-American commodity cultures, 1820–1939
Claire L. Jones (ed.)

Destigmatising mental illness? Professional politics and public education in Britain, 1870–1970
Vicky Long

Intellectual disability: a conceptual history, 1200–1900
Patrick McDonagh, C. F. Goodey and Tim Stainton (eds)

Fools and idiots? Intellectual disability in the Middle Ages
Irina Metzler

Framing the moron: the social construction of feeble-mindedness in the American eugenics era
Gerald V. O'Brien

Recycling the disabled: army, medicine, and modernity in WWI Germany
Heather R. Perry

Shell-shocked British Army veterans in Ireland, 1918-39: A difficult homecoming
Michael Robinson

Disability in the Industrial Revolution: Physical impairment in British coalmining, 1780–1880
David M. Turner and Daniel Blackie

Worth saving: disabled children during the Second World War
Sue Wheatcroft

ERADICATING DEAFNESS?

GENETICS, PATHOLOGY, AND DIVERSITY IN TWENTIETH-CENTURY AMERICA

Marion Andrea Schmidt

Manchester University Press

Copyright © Marion Andrea Schmidt 2020

The right of Marion Andrea Schmidt to be identified as the author of this work has been asserted by her in accordance with the Copyright, Designs and Patents Act 1988.

Published by Manchester University Press
Oxford Road, Manchester M13 9PL

www.manchesteruniversitypress.co.uk

British Library Cataloguing-in-Publication Data
A catalogue record for this book is available from the British Library

ISBN 978 1 5261 3817 0 hardback
ISBN 978 1 5261 8239 5 paperback

First published 2020

The publisher has no responsibility for the persistence or accuracy of URLs for any external or third-party internet websites referred to in this book, and does not guarantee that any content on such websites is, or will remain, accurate or appropriate.

Typeset in 10/12pt Arno Pro by
Servis Filmsetting Ltd, Stockport, Cheshire

Contents

List of figures	page vi
Series editors' foreword	vii
Acknowledgements	viii
A note on terminology	ix
Introduction: of races and genocides	1
1 The sciences of deafness: deaf people as objects of research, reform, and eugenics, 1900–1940	17
2 Concerned and puzzled: heredity research and counselling at the Clarke School, 1930–1960	43
3 Minorities and pathologies: psychogenetic counselling at the New York State Psychiatric Institute, 1955–1969	71
4 Preventing tragedy, negotiating normalcy: the changing meaning of Usher syndrome, 1960–1980	107
5 Signing risk and chance: collaborating for culturally sensitive counselling, 1970–1990	138
Conclusion: from Bell to biodiversity	166
Bibliography	179
Index	198

Figures

1. Postcard of Hubbard Hall, Clarke School for the Deaf, c. 1920s 29
2. Edna Levine talking at a NYSPI meeting, New York State Psychiatric Institute, 1958 82
3. Project staff learning sign language, New York State Psychiatric Institute, 1958 92
4. Psychiatric interview with a deaf patient, New York State Psychiatric Institute, 1958 93
5. 'Have you ever wondered?', detail from a Gallaudet Genetic Services Center Brochure, c. mid-1990s 158
6. 'Become empowered', detail from a Gallaudet Genetic Services Center Brochure, c. mid-1990s 159

Series editors' foreword

You know a subject has achieved maturity when a book series is dedicated to it. In the case of disability, while it has co-existed with human beings for centuries the study of disability's history is still quite young.

In setting up this series, we chose to encourage multi-methodologic history rather than a purely traditional historical approach, as researchers in disability history come from a wide variety of disciplinary backgrounds. Equally 'disability' history is a diverse topic which benefits from a variety of approaches in order to appreciate its multi-dimensional characteristics.

A test for the team of authors and editors who bring you this series is typical of most series, but disability also brings other consequential challenges. At this time disability is highly contested as a social category in both developing and developed contexts. Inclusion, philosophy, money, education, visibility, sexuality, identity and exclusion are but a handful of the social categories in play. With this degree of politicisation, language is necessarily a cardinal focus.

In an effort to support the plurality of historical voices, the editors have elected to give fair rein to language. Language is historically contingent, and can appear offensive to our contemporary sensitivities. The authors and editors believe that the use of terminology that accurately reflects the historical period of any book in the series will assist readers in their understanding of the history of disability in time and place.

Finally, disability offers the cultural, social and intellectual historian a new 'take' on the world we know. We see disability history as one of a few nascent fields with the potential to reposition our understanding of the flow of cultures, society, institutions, ideas and lived experience. Conceptualisations of 'society' since the early modern period have heavily stressed principles of autonomy, rationality and the subjectivity of the individual agent. Consequently we are frequently oblivious to the historical contingency of the present with respect to those elements. Disability disturbs those foundational features of 'the modern.' Studying disability history helps us resituate our policies, our beliefs and our experiences.

Julie Anderson
Walton O. Schalick, III

Acknowledgements

Over the last eight years, many people have supported my research and have contributed in turning this project into a book. At Johns Hopkins, Nathaniel Comfort patiently listened to first outlines and closely read and advised on many, many drafts. I am also much indebted to Dan Todes for his dedication to teaching, his calming influence, patience, and for many good conversations; and to Jeremy Green for his abilities see the bigger picture when I saw trees rather than the forest. Ronald Walters and Brian Greenwald were my go-to scholars for American and Deaf history, respectively. Cathy Kudlick, my mentor in the AHA disability history mentoring program, has supported my venture into this field and helped me think through questions of disciplinary boundaries. Other scholarly communities in the history of medicine, psychiatry, and disability have helped my growth as a scholar. The AHA disability history reading group in particular provided a lively exchange of thoughts and support. Michelle Spinelli, in particular, patiently read many drafts. Sabine Arnaud at the Max-Planck-Institute für Wissenschaftsgeschichte provided important ties to the history of deafness in Europe, as did Maike Rotzoll and Christian Pross for the history of psychiatry. With Anja Werner I have been in a constant dialogue on deaf history that has helped me put the American case in perspective. I also thank the anonymous reviewer for their very thoughtful and helpful input. Walton Schalick, Emma Brennan, and the team at Manchester University Press were a pleasure to work with.

The help and knowledge of many archivists and librarians have much enriched this book: Christine Ruggere, curator at the JHU Institute of the History of Medicine's Historical Collection, Kathy Lafferty at the University of Kansas Spencer Research Library, Jody Sidklaus at the Rochester Institute for Technology Archives, James Sweatt at the Vanderbilt University Eskind Biomedical Library, the staff at the Gallaudet archives, who patiently put up with my lack of signing skills, and Danielle Kovacs at Umass Amherst Special Collections, who has been exceptionally dedicated to finding and providing me with the documents I vaguely asked for. Likewise, this book would not have been possible without the willingness of my oral history interview partners to engage in conversation, share their life stories, and reflect on their scientific practices.

My family and friends in Baltimore, Mississippi, and Portland, the Black Forest, Freiburg, Paderborn, Gießen, and Berlin provided me with support and food, access to kids and cats, American Thanksgivings and Spring Breaks, and reason to travel all over. Jonas I thank for his love and support and music.

A note on terminology

The historical actors in this book use contemporary terms that are now considered offensive or derogatory, such as 'degenerate', 'feeble-minded', or 'retarded'. Where it makes sense, I have replaced these terms with more neutral terminology, otherwise I have used quotation marks.

This book also engages with the changing meaning of what is considered 'normal' (from passing as hearing or non-disabled to considering deafness as part of being normal), as well as with the scholarly literature on normalization, normalcy, and deviance in the history of science, medicine, and disability. While the historical usage of 'normal' is marked with quotation marks, the analytical terminology is not.

INTRODUCTION:
OF RACES AND GENOCIDES

Today, Alexander Graham Bell is most famous for his invention of the telephone. In his time, however, he was also known as a eugenicist and as a highly influential figure in deaf education. These combined interests in eugenics and education led him to look into the marriage patterns of deaf people and whether their children were hearing or deaf. He studied census data and records from residential schools, where at the time most deaf children were educated. These schools also were centres of flourishing deaf communities, with their own clubs, churches, and newspapers, and their own language, American Sign Language (ASL). However, what for deaf people was a cherished community, for Bell was reason for concern. In 1883, he presented the results of his research in a speech to the US National Academy of Sciences, titled *Memoir Upon the Formation of a Deaf Variety of the Human Race*. He believed that educating deaf children in these residential, sign-language schools isolated them from hearing society. Even more so, it encouraged them to find their future spouses within this group, entering a marriage in which they might pass on deafness to their children. There was then, in Bell's nineteenth-century understanding of heredity, the danger of a social issue becoming a biological problem: if deaf people continued to marry each other, they would increase the occurrence of deafness. In the long term, he warned, this might even, 'through a number of successive generations', result in a 'deaf variety of the human race'. Such a 'defective race of human beings', he believed, 'would be a great calamity to the world'.[1]

In 2003, over a century after Bell's *Memoir*, American geneticist Walter Nance confirmed Bell's fears, in a modernized way. By the early 2000s, geneticists had identified several hundred different genes involved in hearing loss. Some of these are very rare, others more common. And there was one recessive form – connexin 26 or *GJB2* deafness – that accounts for about half of all genetic cases in the US. Connexin 26 is a protein that allows ions and molecules to pass between cells and is necessary for hearing. If a non-working gene sequence coding for it – *GJB2* – is passed on by both parents, this results in congenital, sensoneural deafness. Apparently, however, this particular form had not always been so frequent. Rather, Nance found that over the course of the last 200 years, the frequency of connexin 26 deafness had increased in the US because deaf people often married each other. Like Bell, Nance believed that the establishment of residential deaf schools during the nineteenth century, and, in turn, the development of deaf communities and identities, played a role, providing a marriage pool of people from the same sociolinguistic background. Nance, however, found nothing reprehensible about this development. As a geneticist, he was familiar with the fact that individuals often marry within their own sociocultural group, and saw no difference in deaf people doing so, too. 'Unless we are also prepared to abolish racial and ethnic homogamy', he wrote, 'there would appear to be no rational genetic basis for prohibiting marriages among the deaf'. Moreover, where Bell had feared the creation of a deaf race, Nance feared that modern biomedicine might threaten the future of deaf culture and community. He asked: will 'future critics view this [development] as one of the medical triumphs of the 21st Century, or as an egregious example of cultural genocide?'[2]

Deafness remains a highly polarizing trait. Roughly, opinions fall into the two camps just sketched out: deafness as a severe disability that is to be prevented and cured (the medical-pathological model), or deafness as the valued trait of a cultural and linguistic community worth preserving (the sociocultural minority model). The latter is now often denoted with a capital D.[3] Probably more than in any other country, sign language, Deaf culture, and community have become visible and accepted in American society. At the same time, however, the counter-narrative of deafness as a defect to be overcome or eradicated remains strong, fuelled by the possibilities and promises of biomedicine and technology. As Kristen C. Harmon puts it, the 'notion of a deaf child who effectively grows up to become hearing is a compelling cultural fantasy'.[4] It is an ideal that puts the strain of passing as 'normal' solely on the shoulders of the deaf person, disregarding the fact that oral communication is an interactive process that can only succeed if hearing people modify their behaviour as well.

When it comes to the highly politicized issue of family and reproduction, there are, apparently, clear limits to what kind of deaf difference is considered acceptable. To many hearing people, the notion that deaf parents might not care whether their child is deaf or hearing, or might even prefer a deaf child, remains strange, disturbing, and incomprehensible. Many American geneticists, on the other hand, have not only come to accept this preference, but embrace it. Walter Nance, for example, explained already in 1977 that he 'would certainly respect the right of a deaf couple to want a deaf child'. In such a situation, the geneticist could even 'help them select a partner' that would increase the likelihood of such an outcome.[5]

Nance is far from a marginal figure in American genetics. Apart from being an internationally renowned expert on genetic deafness, he has been eminent in twin research and linkage studies, co-authoring over 300 publications. He headed the Virginia Commonwealth College's Department of Human Genetics from 1975 to 2002, was president of the American Board of Medical Genetics in 1986, president of the American Society of Human Genetics (ASHG) in 1992, and received the ASHG leadership award for his mentoring of a younger generation of geneticists in 2007. Since the 1970s, Nance and others have developed a culturally sensitive form of genetic counselling that stresses the need for communication in sign language and for non-judgemental attitudes. This is not a development limited solely to the US. In the UK, geneticist Anna Middleton has conducted extensive research on deaf people's reproductive preferences, and has promoted a transcultural approach to genetic counselling.[6]

How, then, did we go from Bell to Nance, from considering deafness a grave pathology and deaf people's reproductive habits a threat to considering biomedical technology a threat to Deaf culture? And why do some (hearing) professionals side with Deaf culture while others take a medical-pathological approach? This is the topic of this book. I trace how perceptions of deafness and deaf people evolved in the US from the late nineteenth to the late twentieth century, how these perceptions shaped genetic deafness research, what goals researchers pursued, and how they interacted with their patients and objects of research. How did scientists justify their intervention in the private matters of marriage, family life, and reproduction? What rights, autonomy, and capability did they grant to deaf people, how did they react to 'deviant' perspectives, non-conforming with expectations about how a deaf person should behave? What needed to happen to turn such miscommunication and mismatched expectations into an exchange of opinions, and how did this change the role of scientists, lay people and activists?

This is thus also a history of the relationship between different deaf and medical-scientific communities – a relationship that has long been marked by mutual distrust and preconceptions. In Deaf history, it is often rendered as a story of oppressing sign language and deaf culture under the umbrella of making deaf people 'normal'.[7] Medical and scientific communities, on the other hand, are still often perplexed by the existence of Deaf identities, and concerned about their 'resistance' to interventions aiming to cure deafness.[8]

This book chronicles this disconnect between hearing professionals and the deaf people who were the targets of their science. For a long time, this was, indeed, a sharp and anxiously guarded divide. During the first half of the twentieth century, it was almost exclusively hearing professionals who conducted research, relegating deaf people to being patients, service recipients, or objects of research. With a combination of paternalistic assumptions and purposeful ignorance, deaf perspectives thus were systematically excluded from science and medicine. It was only in the 1950s that this almost absolute division slowly began to unravel, with genetic deafness research – perhaps surprisingly – at the forefront of professionals working with deaf communities.

Standing at the intersection between Deaf and disability history and the history of science and medicine, this book thus looks at how predominantly hearing professionals have researched hereditary deafness and interacted with deaf people, and at the heredity counselling they gave. This focus on professional perspectives and practices has pragmatic reasons – as a hearing historian, I focus on the sources accessible to me and leave an in-depth exploration of deaf people's experience with genetics to someone better suited for this task.[9] I also believe, however, that looking at the mechanisms of oppressing and eradicating deaf perspectives, and, respectively, of inclusion and diversification is a crucial contribution to both Deaf history and to a cultural history of biomedicine. When Douglas Baynton remarked about his history of sign language that it was 'chiefly a history of hearing people', in which a majority makes decisions for a minority,[10] this is true to a good extent for this book, too. Yet reading against the grain of professional perspectives, it is also a story of deaf people's perseverance in maintaining their culture, language, and identity, and, from the 1950s onward, of a growing interest among hearing professionals in learning more about this culture and identity.

Looking at such patterns of exclusion and diversification is not just a matter of history. Analysing how exclusion and diversification worked in the past helps us understand why, in the present, some fields and professions perceive deafness as valuable difference and others perceive it as something to be normalized. Through examples of the various disciplines involved in hereditary deafness research and counselling, I thus offer a corrective to the still prevailing trend in Deaf and disability history to see in science and medicine forces that have uniformly pathologized disability. The history of genetic deafness research shows a messier and more complicated trajectory. It makes visible, for example, the 1950's roots of a social model of disability in the social sciences, or the confluence of biomedicalization with late twentieth-century activist policies that emphasize biodiversity and – in some form or other – biological essentialism.[11]

Hereditary deafness research was never an isolated enterprise. It has occupied eugenicists and geneticists, educators and psychologists, physicians, audiologists, and public health officials, all of whom had distinct beliefs about who and what deaf people could and should be. Such beliefs reflected larger and changing ideals about citizenship, body and mind, individual and society. Into the nineteenth century, deafness and disability were mainly matters of charity, education, and religion. By the late nineteenth century, however, science and medicine gained unprecedented power as drivers of modernization, of bringing into line the individual with the ideal of modern, bourgeois, and capitalistic citizenship. With deafness, too, by the late nineteenth century, various sciences had become engaged in the process of identifying what, in the first place, made deaf people different, in order for these differences to be eradicated or normalized. This could take the form of preventing or treating conditions causing hearing loss, or of various social-educational reforms based on the belief that deaf people were capable of living as almost-hearing in hearing society. Hereditary deafness research took place in this larger narrative of progress through science. It simultaneously promised uplift through normalization and pathologized and marginalized visible displays of deafness.[12]

Education played a key role in this endeavour, and it was closely tied to eugenic beliefs. In the late nineteenth century, A. G. Bell was the most prominent advocate of oralism, the practice of teaching deaf people speech and lip-reading. He strongly opposed the then predominant use of sign language – also called manualism – as isolating. Although long considered the most effective teaching tool and a legitimate language of its own, sign language, and with it signing deaf communities, came under suspicion by the late nineteenth century. Darwinism and evolutionary thought played a key role. In an evolutionary framework, sign language was no longer a God-given, natural language, but placed low on the evolutionary ladder, somewhere between gesticulating apes and 'savages'. Oralism, on the other hand, promised to uplift the deaf child into a state of full humanity and civilization.[13]

For Bell, oralism was not only an educational tool, but also the answer to the problem of deaf intermarriage. Enabling deaf people to speak would end their separatism and integrate them into hearing society. It would discourage deaf intermarriage and thus avert the danger of a deaf race. Bell's combination of oralism and eugenics shaped both the course of deaf education and of heredity research from the 1880s to at least the 1950s, instilling in professionals a persistent fear that deaf people's 'deviant' marriage habits would lead to an increase in deafness. Vice versa, the Deaf community and Deaf history remember Bell's *Memoir* as a notorious example of the oppressing power of science, yielded by hearing society to eradicate deaf difference.[14]

Hereditary deafness research thus is part of the larger history of eugenics and genetics. Historians have long debated whether and when eugenics ended, and whether and how much current medical genetics is rooted in eugenic thought and principles. Some have portrayed eugenics as a biased pseudo-science, unlike modern genetics, which is grounded in facts and pursues the noble goal of eradicating suffering, disease, and disability. This is a narrative embraced and actively put forward by geneticists themselves since the 1940s.[15] A younger generation of historians have criticized and deconstructed this idealization. Looking beyond classical studies of laboratories and legislation to a wider set of beliefs, practices, and populations, they have pointed to the enduring influence of eugenic thought, for example in mid-century notions of gender and marriage, the pro-natalist idealization of the middle-class family, and not least the sterilization of women of colour, from native or minority communities, or with disabilities, which went on in many countries at least into the 1970s, if not the present.[16]

What becomes clear in this newer work is the allure eugenics had to many contemporary health and reform movements as an instrument of social reform itself. Like many of these movements – including school reform and deaf education – eugenics had at its core the creation of a modern, progressive, and productive citizen. It operated between the poles of normalizing those supposedly capable of becoming such a citizen, and of 'defending' society from the 'deviant' groups whose inferiority was supposedly inborn and beyond saving by social reform: individuals with physical or intellectual disabilities, racial or ethnic minorities, immigrants from 'undesirable' countries, or migrant workers were all seen as a threat to the 'healthy' nation.[17] The history of genetic deafness is part of this larger history of social and public health reform, of turning the 'worthy' disabled into good, productive citizens, and of excluding those who did not fit those ideals. In their embrace of eugenics as an instrument of betterment, teachers for the deaf pursued a precarious policy claiming that deaf people were unlike the 'feeble-minded' targeted by coercive sterilization legislation. Instead, they aimed to instil in deaf students a sense for eugenically 'responsible' marriages – that is, to hearing people.

The history of genetic deafness blurs the lines between eugenics and medical genetics by exposing changing and divergent definitions of disability. Medical genetics rose to prominence not least because it promised to eradicate disability and suffering (a promise still largely unfulfilled).[18] Disability scholars have long questioned the ableist assumptions in this automatic equation of disability and suffering. They have pointed instead to underlying fears and preconceptions that drive the desire to eradicate or make invisible disability and otherness. To understand these preconceptions, we must look at who was considered disabled at various points in time, across cultures, economic systems, and religious beliefs. Thus, the experience of being deaf and how society perceived deaf people have varied widely – to the point that sometimes they were not considered disabled at all. These sociocultural or sociolinguistic models of understanding disability and deafness have been at the centre of academic Deaf and disability studies, and have provided a solid base for activists who have been challenging bias, discrimination, and exclusion. Consequently, the origins of sociocultural models have usually been placed with the Deaf and disability activism of the 1960s, 1970s, and 1980s, and the academization of Deaf and disability studies from the 1990s onwards.[19]

The period from the 1940s to the 1960s, on the other hand, is often still treated as an in-between period, bridging the oppressive medicalization of the first half of the twentieth century and its repudiation by activists towards its end. I argue, however, that it is just in these mid-century decades that we can find early roots of sociocultural models of deafness and disability, which have been mostly overlooked so far, but which were crucial for reorienting professional perspectives in genetic deafness research and other fields. In the 1950s, sociologists, psychologists, and rehabilitation workers began looking at the experiences of deaf or disabled individuals with the lens of contemporary social research: an interest in the nature of discrimination and bias, majority–minority relations, family, identity, and selfhood. To be sure, these approaches usually were more ambivalent than current sociocultural models of disability – yet it is exactly this meandering between delineating pathology and sociocultural difference that complicates our understanding of Deaf and disability history. Looking at the origins and development of sociocultural models also reminds us that these models are not absolute, but that they emerged under specific and ever-changing historic circumstances.

Genetic deafness research seems like an unlikely field for these new approaches to play out – yet from the 1950s on, genetic deafness researchers were at the forefront of looking at genetic counselling from a psychosocial angle. The 1950s and 1960s were the time in which medical genetics matured as an independent discipline at universities and hospitals, part of the general rapid growth of large-scale, laboratory-reliant biomedicine. It was a time of immense progress in understanding genetic mechanisms, and of a resulting optimism about defining and treating genetic conditions. It was also a time of a rhetorical, if not necessarily ideological, reorientation. As geneticists turned to the 'normal' middle-class family, they embraced non-directive, client-centred counselling as their main tool. This turn towards non-directive counselling facilitated an interest in better understanding – and manipulating – patients' emotional processes in learning about a disability or genetic condition in themselves, their family, or child. Interest in these psychosocial dimensions of genetic counselling and awareness did not necessarily change or negate eugenic thought. As Alexandra Stern or Molly Ladd-Taylor have shown, the psychosocial genetic counselling that emerged in the late 1940s actually reinforced conservative gender and family norms, and tended to exclude children with disabilities from the idealized 'normal' family. Yet, as I argue through the example of deafness, it also increasingly left decisions of what was a 'normal' family to the client, and thus allowed for more individualized, relativistic, and sociocultural definitions of disability and normalcy.[20]

This psychosocial approach coincided with and helped along a larger shift in geneticists' goals: from the very specific goal of preventing certain hereditary conditions they came to emphasize the importance of genetic self-knowledge for modern citizens, who should decide for themselves what this knowledge meant. These sociocultural and psychosocial models influenced genetics from the 1950s on, tempering and at the same time reinforcing biologistic thought. They imbued genetic knowledge with a new sense of identity that relativized clean-cut definitions of pathology and social worth, yet strengthened the notion that genetic awareness was a crucial skill for navigating the risks and potentials of modern life. Genetic deafness research in the second half of the twentieth century cannot be separated from these changes, which facilitated new forms of interaction between geneticists and patient communities.

The history of genetic deafness research also complicates narratives of scientific progress. It illuminates the enduring gap between the promises and the realities of genetics, between knowledge – or the lack thereof – and its applications. Rather than linear progress, or a clean-cut relationship between knowing and doing, it reveals, instead, a certain irony. During the first half of the twentieth century, contemporary understandings of heredity could not account for the immense complexity and diversity of hereditary deafness – today, we know of more than 100 genes causing non-syndromic hearing loss, and more than 400 syndromes involving hearing loss.[21] To researchers in the 1920s, 1930s, and 1940s, looking for simple Mendelian patterns, it remained a puzzling and unpredictable phenomenon. Yet despite – or just because of – the inability to predict whether somebody was genetically deaf or would have deaf children, professionals across different fields agreed that deaf people should not marry each other. This consensus would dissolve when, by the 1960s, geneticists became more confident about their diagnosis and prognosis – and as they developed a more diverse understanding of what it meant to be deaf.

There was then, not only a disconnection between professionals and deaf people, but increasingly also between different fields concerned with different aspects of deafness. Where geneticists stood depended not only on the internal paradigms of their field, but also on with whom they collaborated. Over the course of the twentieth century, they worked with oralist educators or audiologists and with psychologists and psychiatrists primarily interested in the psychosocial dimensions of deafness; within institutions aiming at curing and eradicating deafness, or with d/Deaf individuals, professionals or communities who introduced researchers to their language and culture. Such interdisciplinary alliances formed what Ludwik Fleck called thought collectives, specific beliefs about the nature of deafness.[22] These 'thought collectives' shaped and circumscribed how professionals perceived deaf people, and how new research was incorporated into existing bodies of knowledge – or was ignored or rejected as irrelevant, ideological, or unscientific. They offered different ways of justifying research and professional intervention into matters of marriage, family, and reproduction, ranging from preventing disability to promoting diversity, health care justice, and minority identities.

Organization and chapter overview

To those interested in changing definitions of pathology, diversity, scientific progress, and reproductive responsibility, the history of genetic deafness offers a great advantage. It was a rather small field, yet its actors and institutions also were influential leaders in their respective disciplines: deaf education and activism, eugenics and genetics, psychology and psychiatry. The following chapters thus are a series of interrelated case studies of these main locations and protagonists of genetic deafness research, moving chronologically from the 1920s to the 1990s. Each chapter addresses how a set of professionals approached the 'problem' of hereditary deafness within a certain institution or context, and how they perceived deaf people as recipients of charity, educational uplift, medical or professional intervention, as objects of, or partners in, research.

Chapter 1 introduces one such pivotal location, the Clarke School for the Deaf in Northampton, Massachusetts. Founded in 1867 as the first permanent oralist school in the US, and soon the most influential such institution, it promised to give speech to deaf children, and thus turn them into productive and responsible citizens. This chapter will look at how heredity research and eugenics became part of the school's mission with the establishment of a research department in 1928. Here, in the wake of A. G. Bell's *Memoir*, oralism formed a long-lasting alliance with eugenics. It was based on the apparent truism that it was best if deaf people did not marry each other, both so they would not pass on their 'defect' to future generations and so that they would assimilate into hearing society. To the outside, then, the school presented a triumphant story of 'normalizing' deaf children via science and hard work.[23] Yet a closer look at the school's research department, with its contribution from outside researchers, reveals a microcosm of differing professional approaches to deafness, with overlaps, fissions, and disconnect to the school's oralism. Psychologists Fritz and Grace Moore Heider, for example, produced at Clarke the first psychosocial study of the signing deaf community as a social minority.

This diversification of beliefs and approaches also is important in Chapter 2, which focuses on hereditary deafness research and counselling at the Clarke School from the 1930s to the 1960s. These decades span the period from state-driven eugenics to the establishment of modern medical genetics, with immense changes in understanding heredity. Human heredity research in the 1920s and 1930s was mainly a matter of collecting traits and medical information in order to find dominant or recessive patterns – a task for which the Clarke School was perfectly suited. With a large student body plus their families at hand, they collected pedigrees, medical, and audiological information. With their research and publications, the school became a leading centre of hereditary deafness research – at least for a while. This was not least because it collaborated with some of the leading figures and institutions of eugenics and genetics, including the Eugenic Record Office (ERO) in the 1930s and the National Institutes of Health (NIH) in the 1960s. These collaborations between an oralist school and outside researchers once again make visible different beliefs about what research should achieve and what deafness was, how to do heredity counselling, and the degree of reproductive agency that should be granted to deaf people. Ironically, it was geneticists' increasingly sophisticated understanding of hereditary mechanisms that lead to an unravelling of their alliance with oralist educators in the 1960s: increasingly confident that deaf couples could have a 'normal' family – that is, one without a deaf child – they no longer discouraged deaf intermarriage per se. Oralist educators, on the other hand, still considered it a failure of assimilation to hearing society.

Chapter 3 will leave the Clarke School behind and move to another pivotal institution of genetic deafness research, the New York State Psychiatric Institute (NYSPI). Here, psychiatric geneticist Franz Kallmann and his co-workers developed the first specialized psychiatric and genetic counselling services for deaf people. They began offering services in sign language in a time in which the vast majority of professionals still vehemently rejected signing. Realized in close collaboration with the New York State deaf community, the project was a highly influential turning point in how deaf people were perceived in science, in the design of services serving them, and in the goals pursued in genetic deafness research. It reveals a surprising confluence of eugenic thought, the social sciences, and psychiatric reform in mid-century projects aimed at improving health care services for 'neglected' minorities. Genetic counselling, the NYSPI researchers claimed, was such a health service, and deaf people were entitled to it, just like any other citizen. This, I argue, was part of a larger turn in Cold War America towards depicting genetics as democratic science that enabled, rather than restricted, 'normal', happy, and well-adjusted family life. Genetic information was to be essential knowledge to forming such a family. In this context, it was no longer primarily deafness that was to be prevented, but potential psychosocial 'maladjustment' that might – or might not – result from it.

Negotiations over what was pathological and should be prevented by which means are also at the core of Chapter 4. It contrasts eugenic campaigns to prevent Usher syndrome – congenital deafness and progressive vision loss – with the lived experience of deaf-blind people, and the way they changed the conversation about their capabilities and life trajectories. These debates during the 1970s and 1980s bring up themes that are still prevalent today in talking about scientific progress, bioethics, and disability. In the 1950s and 1960s, rapid advances in genetics made it possible to identify an ever-growing number of subforms of genetic deafness. This progress brought with it the hope that soon geneticists would also be able to cure the underlying biochemical defects. These hopes, however, never manifested, and thus, genetic counselling and 'therapeutic abortion' remained (and to this day usually remain) the main avenue of prevention. This is a familiar story, then. Yet with Usher syndrome, it comes with a twist that shows how closely aligned eugenic motives and activism, ableism and advocacy can be. By the late 1960s, a growing number of professionals had come to embrace a sociocultural minority model of deafness, seeing themselves as deaf people's allies in advocating for sign language and Deaf culture. These same professionals, however, considered deaf-blindness among the worst, most tragic disabilities imaginable – a perspective they shared with many deaf people. And so, with Usher syndrome, it seemed ethically and economically right to invest in eugenic prevention rather than in improving lives that seemed hardly worth living. Deaf-blind patient activists, however, would challenge this dehumanizing position and shifted the conversation towards fighting against bias and discrimination and improving access to education and services. Their negotiation of deaf-blind identity points to still underexplored overlaps between deaf and disability movements and communities.

Chapter 5 looks once more at what happened when geneticists encountered opinions that contradicted their own perceptions of deafness and genetic prevention. By example of the careers of Walter Nance, and his students and co-workers Joann Boughman and Kathleen Arnos, I explore what it took for geneticists to move from a medical-pathological to a sociocultural model of deafness; and what they gained from aligning themselves with the one or the other. Committed to non-directive, client-centred counselling, they believed that working with Deaf communities was integral to making genetic counselling accessible and acceptable. By the 1970s and 1980s, such 'genetic communities', or alliances between geneticists and target populations, had become common, forming, for example, around conditions such as Tay-Sachs syndrome or Chorea Huntington, or, indeed, Usher syndrome.[24] Usually, however, they worked towards finding a cure, better prevention, or other medical solutions. Nance and his co-workers, on the other hand, tried to find a form of genetic counselling that was not threatening to Deaf identities, reframing, for example, the 'risk' of having a deaf child into a 'chance'.

Consequently, the Gallaudet Genetic Services Center, established in 1984 in the heart of American Deaf culture and community, acknowledged deafness as a 'normal', even desirable trait, and promoted genetic self-awareness as an 'empowering' tool in Deaf people's struggle for recognition and acceptance. In doing so, I argue, it precipitated and helped prepare the late twentieth-century merger of cultural and biological diversity. When, in recent years, Deaf and disability activists have replaced the notion of defective genes with the more inclusive message of biodiversity, this is not a simple process of reclaiming knowledge from the pathologizing realms of science and medicine. Rather, it is a reclaiming actively encouraged by geneticists, part of a larger psychologization of genetic knowledge and identities that already started in the 1950s. A history of genetic deafness thus also is a cultural history of citizenship and identity politics, and of health professionals embracing health and disability activism as part of professional identity. Surveying these developments, it provides a deeper understanding of current discussions about the promises and limits of biomedicine, about reproductive choice, bioethics, and disability.

Notes

1 A. G. Bell, *Memoir Upon the Formation of a Deaf Variety of the Human Race* (Washington, DC: U.S. Government Printing Office, 1884), http://catalog.hathitrust.org/api/volumes/oclc/2141276.html [accessed 16 October 2019], pp. 4, 41.

2 W. E. Nance, 'The genetics of deafness', *Mental Retardation and Developmental Disabilities Research Reviews*, 9 (2003), 109–19, here 109, 116. Also see W. E. Nance and M. J. Kearsey, 'Relevance of connexin deafness (DFNB1) to human evolution', *American Journal of Human Genetics*, 74:6 (2004), 1081–7. For a

current overview of forms of genetic deafness see A. E. Shearer, M. S. Hildebrand, and R. J. H. Smith, 'Deafness and hereditary hearing loss overview', *NCBI Gene Reviews*, 1999, updated 27 July 2017, www.ncbi.nlm.nih.gov/books/NBK1434 [accessed 30 August 2018].

3 This is a recent convention, suggested in 1972 by linguist James Woodward. I will use Deaf for the time period in the later twentieth century when actors used it themselves, and when the identities in question are sufficiently clear and unambiguous.

4 K. C. Harmon, 'Growing up to become hearing: dreams of passing in oral deaf education', in J. A. Brune and D. J. Wilson (eds), *Disability and Passing: Blurring the Lines of Identity* (Philadelphia, PA: Temple University Press, 2013), pp. 167–98, here 169. For the negotiations involved in lipreading, see e.g. A. Neugebauer, 'Hab ich das richtig verstanden. Den Möglichkeitsraum eingrenzen. Lippenlesen und Interaktion', in M. Schmidt and A. Werner, *Zwischen Fremdbestimmung und Autonomie Neue Impulse zur Gehörlosengeschichte in Deutschland, Österreich und der Schweiz* (Bielefeld: Transcript, 2019), pp. 119–52.

5 W. E. Nance, S. P. Rose, P. M. Conneally, and J. Z. Miller, 'Opportunities for genetic counseling through institutional ascertainment of affected probands', in H. A. Lubs and F. F. De la Cruz (eds), *Genetic Counseling* (New York: Raven Press, 1977), pp. 307–31, here 331.

6 See e.g. K. S. Arnos, M. Cunningham, J. Israel, and M. L. Marazita, 'Innovative approach to genetic counseling services for the deaf population', *American Journal of Medical Genetics*, 44 (1992), 345–5. For the UK see A. Middleton, F. Robson, L. Burnell, and M. Ahmed, 'Providing a transcultural genetic counseling service in the UK', *Journal of Genetic Counseling*, 16:5 (2007), 567–82; A. Middleton, S. D. Emery, and G. H. Turner, 'Views, knowledge, and beliefs about genetics and genetic counseling among deaf people' *Sign Language Studies*, 10:2 (2010), 170–96.

7 For this perspective see e.g. J. Branson and D. Miller, *Damned for Their Difference: The Cultural Construction of Deaf People as Disabled: A Sociological History* (Washington, DC: Gallaudet University Press, 2002); H. Lane, R. Hoffmeister, and B. J. Bahan, *A Journey into the Deaf-World* (San Diego, CA: DawnSignPress, 1996).

8 Bioethicists, for example, have tried to define disability and suffering by notions of functionality that gloss over sociocultural determinants, individual wishes and circumstances. See J. Glover, *Choosing Children: Genes, Disability, and Design* (Oxford: Clarendon Press, 2006). Blind bioethicist Adrianne Asch on the other hand criticized this functionalist and universalist approach. See e.g. E. Parens and A. Asch, *Prenatal Testing and Disability Rights* (Washington, DC: Georgetown University Press, 2000). For a Deaf studies perspectives see the contributions to J. V. Van Cleve (ed.), *Genetics, Disability, and Deafness* (Washington, DC: Gallaudet University Press, 2004).

9 There is still much to explore on the experiences and attitudes of different groups of

deaf people with eugenics and genetics. For the late nineteenth and early twentieth century see e.g. W. T. Ennis, 'Hereditarian ideas and eugenic ideals at the National Deaf-Mute College' (PhD dissertation, University of Iowa, 2015).

10 D. C. Baynton, *Forbidden Signs: American Culture and the Campaign against Sign Language* (Chicago, IL: University of Chicago Press, 1998), p. 10.

11 For an overview of trends in disability history see e.g. M. Rembis, C. Kudlick, and K. E. Nielsen, 'Introduction', in M. Rembis, C. Kudlick, and K. E. Nielsen (eds), *The Oxford Handbook of Disability History* (New York: Oxford University Press, 2018), pp. 1–18. With these theories, historians of disability and deafness have – implicitly or explicitly – drawn from medicalization theory, which has been advanced in particular by sociologist Peter Conrad. See e.g. P. Conrad, *The Medicalization of Society: On the Transformation of Human Conditions into Treatable Disorders* (Baltimore, MD: Johns Hopkins University Press, 2007).

12 For the transformation of concepts of disability and deafness under the impact of industrialization, modernity and ideals of science and normalization see e.g. D. C. Baynton, '"These pushful days": time and disability in the age of eugenics', *Health and History*, 13:2 (2011), 43–64; L. J. Davis, *Enforcing Normalcy: Disability, Deafness, and the Body* (London: Verso, 1995); L. J. Davis, 'Introduction: disability, normality, and power', in L. J. Davis (ed.), *The Disability Studies Reader* (London; New York: Routledge, 2012), pp. 1–17.

13 The debates over sign language versus oralism belong to the most thoroughly covered topics in Deaf history. For an overview see Baynton, *Forbidden Signs*; R. A. R. Edwards, *Words Made Flesh: Nineteenth-Century Deaf Education and the Growth of Deaf Culture* (New York: New York University Press, 2014).

14 Brian Greenwald has presented the most nuanced study of Bell's educational policies and eugenic research. See B. H. Greenwald, 'Alexander Graham Bell through the lens of eugenics, 1883–1922' (doctoral dissertation, The George Washington University, 2002). Also see J. V. Van Cleve and B. A. Crouch, *A Place of Their Own: Creating the Deaf Community in America* (Washington, DC: Gallaudet University Press, 1989), pp. 142–54; Branson and Miller, *Difference*, pp. 148–54. Next to these academic works, countless blogs and websites recount the tale of A. G. Bell, eugenics and oralism with various degrees of historical accuracy.

15 For this position see e.g. K. M. Ludmerer, *Genetics and American Society: A Historical Appraisal* (Baltimore, MD: Johns Hopkins University Press, 1972); R. S. Cowan, *Heredity and Hope: The Case for Genetic Screening* (Cambridge, MA: Harvard University Press, 2008).

16 For the continuous sterilization of women from minorities see e.g. T. W. Volscho, 'Sterilization racism and pan-ethnic disparities of the past decade: the continued encroachment on reproductive rights', *Wicazo Sa Review*, 25:1 (2010), 17–31; M. C. Gill, *Already Doing It: Intellectual Disability and Sexual Agency* (Minneapolis, MN: University of Minnesota Press, 2015), pp. 105–24; R. M. Kluchin, *Fit to be Tied: Sterilization and Reproductive Rights in America, 1950–1980* (New Brunswick, NJ: Rutgers University Press, 2011), pp. 148–83.

17 I can only point here to a few selected works from this newer historiography of eugenics. For the ties to medicine and public health see in particular D. B. Paul, *Controlling Human Heredity: 1865 to the Present* (Atlantic Highlands, NJ: Humanities Press, 1995); N. C. Comfort, *The Science of Human Perfection: How Genes Became the Heart of American Medicine* (New Haven, CT: Yale University Press, 2012). For the long-lasting influence of eugenics on definitions of gender, family life, and reproduction see e.g. W. Kline, *Building a Better Race: Gender, Sexuality, and Eugenics from the Turn of the Century to the Baby Boom* (Berkeley, CA: University of California Press, 2005); J. Schoen, *Choice & Coercion: Birth Control, Sterilization, and Abortion in Public Health and Welfare* (Chapel Hill, NC: University of North Carolina Press, 2005).

18 See e.g. Cowan, *Heredity and Hope*.

19 I do not intend here to blur the arguments and differences between Deaf and disability history, e.g. the rejection of the label 'disability' by many Deaf people and its active queering and/or appropriation in disability studies. See e.g. C. A. Padden, 'Talking culture: Deaf people and disability studies', *Publications of the Modern Language Association of America*, 120:2 (2005), 508–13; S. Burch and A. Kafer (eds), *Deaf and Disability Studies: Interdisciplinary Perspectives* (Washington, DC: Gallaudet University Press, 2010). For a historiographical overview of disability history see Rembis et al., 'Introduction'; for deafness see e.g. H. Gienow-McConnella, 'The story of Mr. and Mrs. Deaf: Deaf American historiography, past, present, and future', *Critical Disability Discourses/Discourse Critiques dans le Champ du Handicap*, 7 (2015), 109–44.

20 For the origins of non-directive genetic counselling, its psychological dimensions, and reinforcement of gender and family norms see e.g. M. Ladd-Taylor, '"A kind of genetic social work": Sheldon Reed and the origins of genetic counseling', in G. D. Feldberg (ed.), *Women, Health and Nation: Canada and the United States since 1945* (Montreal: McGill-Queen's University Press, 2003), pp. 67–83; A. M. Stern, *Telling Genes: The Story of Genetic Counseling in America* (Baltimore, MD: Johns Hopkins University Press, 2012), in particular pp. 77–90. For the psychologization of genetic information and disability see M. A. Schmidt, 'Birth defects, family dynamics, and mourning loss: psychoanalysis, genetic counseling and disability, 1950–1980', *Psychoanalysis and History*, 21:2 (2019), 147–69.

21 See Shearer et al., 'Deafness and hereditary hearing loss overview'. In current terminology, 'hereditary' and 'genetic' are not necessarily the same, as mutations on the level of gene regions or chromosomes (e.g. with Down Syndrome) can occur anew in each generation. For this book, however, I will follow the contemporary use of historical actors, for which both terms were largely synonymous.

22 L. Fleck, *Entstehung und Entwicklung einer Wissenschaftlichen Tatsache: Einführung in die Lehre vom Denkstil und Denkkollektiv* (Frankfurt am Main: Suhrkamp, 1980 [First edition Basel: Benno Schwabe, 1935]).

23 Today, still, the Clarke School portrays itself as a home-like place, where deaf children thrive and grow into success in hearing society. This narrative has been

challenged by former students, who remember an oppressive atmosphere in which any form of gestural language was punished. Most significant and most recent were accusations of physical and sexual abuse by teacher Mary E. Numbers and her brother during the 1940s, 1950s, and 1960s, which the school confirmed after a 2018 investigation. See e.g. D. Christensen, '"In a glass box": Clarke School for the Deaf alumni detail decades of abuse', *Daily Hampshire Gazette*, 1 January 2019, www.gazettenet.com/Clarke-School-alumni-detail-abuse-they-suffered-19985099 [accessed 29 May 2019].

24 See K. Wailoo, *Dying in the City of the Blues: Sickle Cell Anaemia and the Politics of Race and Health* (Chapel Hill, NC: University of North Carolina Press, 2001); K. Wailoo and S. G. Pemberton, *The Troubled Dream of Genetic Medicine: Ethnicity and Innovation in Tay-Sachs, Cystic Fibrosis, and Sickle Cell Disease* (Baltimore, MD: Johns Hopkins University Press, 2006).

I

THE SCIENCES OF DEAFNESS: DEAF PEOPLE AS OBJECTS OF RESEARCH, REFORM, AND EUGENICS, 1900–1940

In 1927, the Clarke School for the Deaf mobilized their influential contacts to launch a nation-wide fund-raising campaign. The fund was named after the presidential couple, Calvin and Grace Goodhue Coolidge, who had lent their name and support to the campaign. In a period in which disability was often conflated with dangerous degeneracy, the Clarke School convinced prominent donors that deaf children were worth saving by science and progressive reform. While some of the Coolidge Fund went into building maintenance and scholarships, it was also used to establish a small research department with divisions for heredity research, psychology, and phonetics. For the school, these three disciplines stood at the forefront of exploring and ameliorating the effects of deafness, and for thus making deaf education more efficient. The research department was part of the school's holistic mission of uplifting deaf children from their state of 'primitive' speechlessness and turning them into productive, 'almost-normal' citizens who would succeed in hearing society. Next to this educational mission, the school also felt responsible for addressing the 'problem of deafness' more generally, as a matter of public health and prevention. Heredity research and its eugenic application were part of these larger conversations about disability, childhood, and public health, about how to increase the efficiency of education and put science and medicine to 'restoring' the disabled.[1]

If we want to understand how eugenics became part of these conversations, and how it ties in with oralist education, we need to look back at the history of the school, and how deafness and deaf people were treated in science and medicine more generally. In the decades around the turn from the nineteenth to the twentieth century, perceptions of deafness and disability changed profoundly, not least by developments that also ushered in the era of eugenics: the proliferation of evolutionary thought with its impact on classifying humans;

nativist tendencies that redefined American citizenship; the strong belief in science and medicine as powerful instruments of social reform; and, under the influence of industrialization and market capitalism, an equation of individual worth and economic productivity. These developments were marked, simultaneously, by an optimistic belief in uplifting and 'normalizing' people with disabilities via science, charity, and medicine, and by seeing them as portents of moral and social degeneration. In their own ways, both trends were marginalizing. In the age of the paternalistic expert and the social reformer, the individual agency of individuals with disabilities was increasingly limited. Non-conformance with social reform and professional intervention came to be marked as dangerous deviance, as a threat to the social order that often was sanctioned with restricting civil or reproductive rights.[2]

Deafness is a case in point. Whereas in early and mid-nineteenth-century America, deaf culture and communities had flourished relatively unchallenged, they came under close scrutiny in the last third of the century. By the early decades of the twentieth century, a host of different professions – teachers and social workers, physicians of various specializations, public health reformers, and eugenicists – claimed that they knew best how to fix deafness and 'normalize' deaf people. They did not necessarily agree. Research at the Clarke School and their collaboration with outside researchers offers insight to these collaborations and dissonances. In particular, it sheds light on the consensus and alliance between eugenics and oralist education that would shape heredity research in the first half of the twentieth century. When early twentieth-century researchers talked about eugenics, heredity, and deafness, they did so in a framework concerned with the passing on of deafness, but also the standardization and efficiency of education, with mental or social hygiene, childhood studies, or mental testing. In their verdict about various groups of 'defectives', eugenicists drew heavily from psychology, anthropology, medicine, and other disciplines that established physical, intellectual, gender, or moral norms. Placing the Clarke School and its research in a larger framework of social reform and scientific developments, this chapter offers a history of eugenics, disability, and the interdependence between promises of passing as non-disabled on the one hand, and the exclusion of deaf people's perspectives on the other.

The Clarke School for the Deaf: celebrating the uplift of scientific oralism

The Clarke School was founded in 1867 by wealthy New England businessmen as the first permanent school in the US to rely solely on the oral method.

Teaching speech to the deaf was not new per se. It had been the dominant method of deaf education in Germany since the middle of the eighteenth century, and indeed was long known as the 'German' method. The US, however, was influenced by the 'French' or manual method.[3] When state-supported schools for the deaf were founded in the early and mid-nineteenth century, teachers – often deaf themselves – considered sign language the best solution for bringing deaf children within the reach of education and religious salvation. Their goal was for their students to achieve a bilingual mastery of both sign language and (written) English.[4] Sign language also became a defining characteristic of the emerging deaf community. Residential schools for the deaf soon became centres of a flourishing deaf community and culture. Here, deaf children met deaf adults and deaf peers who shared their experiences. They were initiated to sign language, made friends, received an education, moved on, yet stayed in contact with and often married former schoolmates, organized regular social events, or socialized in deaf clubs, churches, and associations. By the 1850s, deaf people formed a subculture and linguistic community similar to those of many immigrant groups.[5]

When, in 1863, five-year-old Mabel Hubbard, daughter of the wealthy Boston lawyer and philanthropist Gardiner Greene Hubbard, fell ill with scarlet fever and lost her hearing, her father had to familiarize himself with the landscape of American deaf education. Fearing that Mabel would lose her speech, he engaged a private tutor and became a well-known advocate of oralist education in Massachusetts. Hubbard's support of oralism was a sign of the time. By the last third of the nineteenth century, sign languages and deaf culture came under close public and scientific scrutiny. As beliefs about humankind and language, disability and medicine, American society and its minorities changed, so did perceptions of deafness, deaf people and their community. Physical and sociocultural normalcy – or at least the appearance thereof – became the new, elusive ideal against which they were measured.[6]

Post-Civil War America came to emphasize the white Anglo-Saxon male as the ideal citizen, and watched its many ethnic and linguistic minorities with suspicion. There were striking similarities in how immigrants, Native Americans, and deaf people were perceived. Not quite taken as full, legitimate citizens yet, they were to leave behind their foreign habits and languages in order to be civilized and uplifted by American values and the English language. The spread of evolutionary thought also had an immense impact. Destroying the God-given division between humans and beasts, Darwinism triggered an anxious search for what distinguished humans from animals. To many, spoken language came to be this distinguishing feature; a reconceptualization with far-reaching consequences for deaf education. As scientists studied gestural communication among animals and 'savage' people, they associated sign language with a lower stage of evolution, in which humans had just barely risen above their primate ancestors. In this new, oralist-evolutionary mind-set, then, failing to master speech signified something more sinister: the inability to overcome the primitive – even savage – state of childhood in order to mature into a fully civilized citizen.[7]

These motives of inspirational uplift, civilization, and normalization also permeated the advocacy of Hubbard and other influential Massachusetts supporters of oralism with whom he soon connected, among them the politician Horace Mann and the educator Samuel Gridley Howe. With extensive fundraising and influential connections, these men finally succeeded in establishing, in 1867, the Clarke Institution for Deaf Mutes in Northampton, with Hubbard as president of the school's corporation. Next to the older, renowned Hartford Asylum, a stronghold of the manual method, Massachusetts now had a second, state-supported oralist school for the deaf. It was named after Northampton businessman John Clarke, who, hard of hearing himself, had donated $50,000. When he died two years later, Clarke made the school a beneficiary in his will, bringing his total donation up to the significant sum of $306,000 – more than any American school for the deaf had ever received up to this point.[8] In 1870, the school board acquired an estate with two houses on Northampton's Round Hill, an idyllic, small town location well-suited to providing, as a school brochure boasted later, as much 'as humanly possible, the warmth of relationship and the natural home atmosphere surrounding the hearing child'.[9]

The school, Schlesinger has pointed out, successfully combined the homely image of a family-like community with that of a daringly progressive institution that challenged tradition.[10] Growing constantly, it soon established a reputation as a pioneer in oralist education. It offered an inspirational story of overcoming disability and becoming fully human through hard work, personal reform, and, not least, through the benefits of scientific progress. With this narrative, it drew from, and significantly contributed to, the story of successful oralist passing as almost-hearing that is still attractive today. Over the next decades, the school would steadily invest time, staff, and resources into researching the different physical, sensory, or psychological dimensions of deafness and their impact on education. Its ties with influential reformers and institutions helped the school in this enterprise. Its connections with Alexander Graham Bell in particular would influence the school's stance on eugenics, hereditary deafness, and oralism.

Oralism, heredity, and deaf intermarriage: A. G. Bell's *Memoir Upon the Formation of a Deaf Variety of the Human Race*

As the inventor of the telephone, Bell is often portrayed as the embodiment of American entrepreneurship; a scientist, self-made man, and philanthropist. In the Deaf community, however, his rejection of sign language and support of eugenics has gained him a much darker reputation. Quite correctly, Deaf scholars have charged him with trying to eliminate two of the pillars of Deaf culture: sign language and residential schools.[11] Bell's science and his life-long advocacy for oralism were inseparable. He was born in Scotland in 1847 into a family occupied with the sciences – and business – of sound and speech. His father Alexander Melville Bell developed Visible Speech, a phonetic system for teaching deaf children spoken language by connecting each sound to a specific, visualized mouth position. Hearing loss also had a personal dimension in the Bell family. Bell's mother Eliza was hard-of-hearing. A painter and musician, she avoided socializing with other deaf people and preferred oral communication. Early on in his career, Bell worked as a teacher for the deaf, tutoring private students. Among them was his future wife, Mabel, whom he met in Northampton, when, in 1876, he travelled to the US to promote his father's system. At the Clarke School, his ideas found a receptive audience. He would remain connected to the school for the rest of his life, and from 1917 to his death in 1922, served as president of the school board. In this function and as a prominent advocate for oralism, he became the school's revered founding figure.[12]

Like many of his contemporaries, Bell was interested in questions of heredity and evolution, both in theory and applied to the better breeding of animals – and humans. In the 1880s, he began studying the marriage patterns of deaf people. Martha's Vineyard, which had an unusually high incidence of deafness, attracted his attention, and he went there to study families with deaf members and their pedigrees.[13] In 1883, he presented the results in a talk to the US National Academy of Sciences, and published them a year later under the title *Memoir Upon the Formation of a Deaf Variety of the Human Race*. Rather than talking about the recently invented telephone, Bell chose a topic that fascinated him and many of his contemporaries: how did the phenomena of selection and variation influence evolution? Deaf people, he pointed out, were an excellent example to study this question because they tended to marry each other in a form of 'continuous selection'. Appealing to larger scientific interests, he thus set up deaf intermarriage as a natural experiment. Investigating whether they passed on deafness to their children would answer the question of whether 'the human race' was 'susceptible of variation by selection'. Bell believed that his data provided a positive answer: it proved that deaf people passed on their deafness, that their intermarriage increased the occurrence of deafness, and that consequently humans were susceptible to selective variation. In turn, his conclusion provided proof of the dangers of this practice: 'the intermarriage of congenital deaf-mutes through a number of successive generations', he claimed, 'should result in the formation of a deaf variety of the human race'. Such a 'defective race of human beings', he warned, 'would be a great calamity to the world'.[14]

The tendency for intermarriage, Bell claimed, was the result of educational intervention. It resulted from educating deaf children at residential schools, effectively separating them from their families and society at large. Schools for the deaf, he lamented, had produced numerous incentives that encouraged deaf people to socialize among each other rather than with the hearing, such as reunions, societies and conventions, newspapers and periodicals. This segregation, he asserted, had supported the most powerful instrument of preventing interaction with hearing society: 'the evolution of a special language' – sign language – 'adapted for the use of such a race'.[15] Portraying late nineteenth-century deaf culture and community as an unintended and tragic biological aberration, Bell thus tapped into contemporary fears about the destructive effects of civilization. His alarm over racial separation and 'class-feeling among the deaf and dumb' mirrored fears of an American society increasingly divided by class, culture, and race in a time of rapid social change, mass immigration, and industrialization.[16]

When it came to preventing such a deaf race, Bell preferred educational reform and oralist assimilation over legal action. It was, Brian Greenwald has argued, his personal and professional acquaintance with deaf people – his mother and wife, former students, and business partners – that made him favour a moderate stance, yet also made oralism his prime eugenic tool. He acted as a buffer between the deaf community and more radical eugenicists who favoured coercive methods. 'We cannot dictate to men and women whom they shall marry', he declared, and added that with the current state of knowledge marriage restrictions would prove impractical anyway. Integrating deaf people into day schools and society, and discouraging them from associating with each other would automatically decrease the incidence of harmful deaf intermarriages. As the most widely known expert on deafness of his time, he wielded much influence. His politics of assimilation and education would become the dominant eugenic strategy to prevent hereditary deafness in the following decades.[17]

In the early 1890s, Bell's sheep breeding experiments on his Nova Scotia estate brought him into contact with others interested in breeding and heredity. In particular, he began corresponding with Charles Davenport, the most influential American eugenicist of his time. He soon became active in the emergent eugenic movement, and a charter member of the Eugenics Committee of the American Breeders' Association (ABA). Founded in 1906, it was the first US-American eugenic association. Deaf-mutism was the subject of one of its ten subcommittees, along with 'feeble-mindedness', epilepsy, and sterilization. In 1910, Bell helped Davenport solicit funds for his Eugenics Record Office (ERO), which would soon become the most influential eugenic institution in the US. He later served as chairman of the Eugenics Record Office's Board of Scientific Directors, presiding over distinguished members such as economist Irving Fisher and Johns Hopkins' William H. Welch.[18]

Many of the ERO's causes seemed worthy of support to Bell, for example their call on stricter immigration legislation. He increasingly disapproved, however, of the ERO's methods and its focus on negative and coercive eugenics. Where ERO representatives wanted to restrict eugenically unfavourable marriages, if needed by legislation, he believed in encouraging 'good' marriages – positive eugenics – as the main instrument of the movement. In 1916, he withdrew from his ERO chairmanship, disappointed with the direction eugenic policies had taken there. In particular, he disagreed with the ERO's advocacy for sterilization legislation, a matter pushed strongly by the new director Harry Laughlin, and over the course of the 1920s and 1930s increasingly accepted by American science and society at large.[19]

Fragile normalcy: deafness and deaf people as a target of eugenics

In early twentieth-century America, eugenics was almost universally attractive. In an age that believed in progress through science, social reform and self-improvement, very few groups or individuals totally rejected eugenic thought and goals. Yet what exactly it meant and how it should be pursued varied considerably depending on one's social, political, and professional position. It could be cast as a scientific quest for understanding and manipulating the biological laws governing nature and society; as a branch of medicine or public health; as part of progressive reform; and as a form of moral guidance for modern life, a kind of religion even. More often than not, eugenic thought was used to defend one's own social position and privileges against the perceived threat of supposedly inferior groups who triggered fears of miscegenation and social unrest: immigrants and the racially other, those perceived as physically, intellectually, morally, socially, or sexually deviant. Yet the target populations of eugenic reform were not sharply defined. Who was granted reproductive responsibility and could claim eugenics as a form of self-improvement and self-evolution, and who, on the contrary, was a menace to society was a matter of perspective and negotiation.[20]

For a long time, historians of eugenics have predominantly focused on the ill-defined group of the 'feeble-minded', who, as Allison Carey noted, had 'emerged as one of the principal enemies in the nation's war against population degeneracy and "race suicide"'.[21] When professionals, politicians, journalists, or lay people wrote about the mentally 'degenerate' and 'defective', it was with fear, contempt, and the urgency of impending doom. Supposedly filling up asylums, hospitals, and prisons, and taxing public welfare and bourgeois good will, socially deviant paupers seemed to have evolved into a race of their own, one that was biologically doomed to moral, physical, and mental degeneracy. Worse still, they threatened to overpower society with their unrepressed reproduction. Given this threat, institutionalization and sterilization seemed necessary and appropriate solutions to many. In 1907, Indiana was the first state to pass legislation that allowed the compulsory sterilization of any 'incurable' criminal or 'feeble-minded' inmate of a state institution. By the end of the 1920s, most US states had passed sterilization laws, encouraged by the favourable Supreme Court decision in Buck vs. Bell in 1927. An estimated 60,000 individuals were sterilized under these laws, predominantly in the 1930s, 1940s and 1950s, although sterilization of women of colour, from minority communities and/or with (supposed) intellectual disabilities continued at the very least into the 1970s, if not the present. This history makes clear how much the right to reproductive autonomy remains a privilege tied to gender, race, and social status.[22]

Individuals labelled as 'feeble-minded' thus were affected disproportionally by coercive eugenics, yet the reach of eugenics went far beyond them. They only stood at the far end of a spectrum of groups targeted for conditions considered hereditary to some degree. Whereas physicians and the public agreed that the 'feeble-minded' and 'degenerate' should not reproduce (uncontrolled), this directive was less easily made with other groups, whose conditions presumably had a hereditary component, but who were thought to contribute valuable – and hereditary – traits to society. Contemporary thought on the heredity of genius and insanity – two traits that seemed closely allied – make clear that notions of eugenic worth were not set in stone. Similarly, historian Arleen Tuchman has shown how early twentieth-century notions of diabetes shaped the debate over the benefits and disadvantages of sterilizing diabetics. The common preconception of diabetes-sufferers as predominantly white, educated, and middle class, Tuchman argues, made coercive eugenic measures seem unnecessary. Some physicians even asserted that diabetics' intellectual capabilities and need for extraordinary self-control outweighed the negative diabetes trait when it came to procreation.[23]

The position of deaf people, too, was complicated. In the first third of the twentieth century, when eugenic thought combined with older presumptions about able-bodied (white and male) civic fitness, their civil rights were challenged in a multitude of ways. Marriage and reproduction, eligibility for a driver's licence, or partaking in New Deal programmes were only some of the contested areas. Debates over deaf intermarriage and reproduction in particular intensified again in the 1920s, as eugenic publications indiscriminately included deaf people into the group of 'defectives', and discussed the need for health certificates prior to marriage. The various state sterilization laws did not explicitly include deaf people, yet some still found themselves within their reach. In an era that equated the ability for speech and lip-reading with intelligence, individuals stigmatized as 'oral failures' often found themselves labelled as 'feeble-minded' or 'retarded'.[24]

Unlike the heterogeneous group labelled 'feeble-minded', deaf people, with their local and national organizations, newspapers, and sense of community had a certain amount of lobbying power and social standing. Their organizations advocated – with at least partial success – against being included in measures targeting 'defectives'. Extensive campaigns portrayed deaf people as productive, educated, and patriotic citizens. These campaigns, Susan Burch and Octavian Robinson pointed out, came at the cost of excluding deaf people who, supposedly, did not fit these criteria. Perpetuating contemporary notions of civic fitness, capitalist productivity, and bodily normalcy, the National Association of the Deaf (NAD) carefully policed the public image of deaf people. Publications increasingly emphasized the healthy deaf family that adhered to middle-class standards and – importantly – produced healthy, hearing children. Such politics were revealing for the power structures within the Deaf community. Its leaders usually were white middle-class men (women members were not allowed to vote until 1964; black members first admitted in 1965).[25] They were often late-deafened and carefully distanced themselves, as Robinson put it, from 'people dangerously classified as "other"'[26] – those congenitally deaf, racially other, or multiply disabled. These tensions, to which historians have only recently given attention, challenge the idealized notion of a unified and uniform deaf community.[27]

Eager to prove their own normalcy and worth, deaf people rejected the labels of disability and eugenic defect for their own person, but nevertheless often applied these labels to others within their community – a strategy common among groups targeted by eugenics. Such ableist assumptions found their expression in NAD positions and policies. In 1907, for example, NAD president George Veditz suggested the establishment of a committee tasked with lobbying against any insinuation that the deaf should be grouped with the real targets of eugenic measures. Terminology was another concern of NAD activism, and one where the interests of the signing deaf community overlapped with advocates of oralism. Both camps advocated the use of 'deaf' instead of the older 'deaf and dumb' because of its associations with mental deficiency. In 1920, the NAD passed a resolution that spoke out against marriages of two congenitally deaf persons. The NAD thus pursued, as Susan Burch put it, a policy of 'personal persuasion over litigation'.[28] Deaf people, the message implied, did not need outside interference to comply with the ideals of good (eugenic) citizenship. To many deaf people, as to their hearing contemporaries, eugenics was an attractive means of social reform. If such scientific reform required some people to relinquish some of their rights and freedoms, this was taken as an unfortunate yet necessary sacrifice for the bigger good – as long as oneself was not affected.[29]

Educators for the deaf, too, distanced their students from any association with 'defectives' and 'degenerates', and in doing so perpetuated beliefs about social deviance and (un)worthiness. A 1919 report by the Conference of Superintendents and Principals of American Schools for the Deaf, for example, confirmed common prejudice, and clad it in new, scientific-progressive terminology. Titled *Standardization, Efficiency, Heredity*, the report picked up on general sentiments among educators and reformers, warning that 'today we are facing the greatest question ever presented to our social life – that of abnormal mentality and feeblemindedness ... which are filling our public schools, our custodial institutions, and our general life, with socially unfit and defective classes'. Deaf people, however, the report insisted repeatedly, did not generally belong to this group. Associating deaf people with the intellectually and morally 'deficient' and 'defectives' was 'ridiculous' and inflicted 'upon the deaf ... an unnecessary brand'. On the contrary, schools for the deaf turned their students into citizens who with their hard work and high morals were America's 'bulwark of liberty'.[30]

Distancing deaf students from those with (supposed) intellectual disabilities was part of the larger stratification of special education during the first decades of the twentieth century. Eugenic thought and prejudice played a significant role in this process. Both schools for the deaf and the 'feeble-minded' had been founded with a shared belief in the power of education to reform the individual, and to restore people with disabilities to social participation and economic usefulness. By the 1910s and 1920s, however, educators and researchers increasingly talked about people with intellectual disabilities in the eugenic language of innate hopelessness. Psychologist Henry Herbert Goddard's famous – and defaming – *The Kallikak Family: A Study in the Heredity of Feeble-Mindedness* (1912) is just one notorious example for the close ties between contemporary psychology, eugenics, and education. Goddard was a well-respected psychologist who played a crucial role in introducing and promoting intelligence testing in the US. For Goddard, as for many of his contemporaries, social deviance and intellectual inferiority were really a matter of biology, the inherent traits of a hopelessly 'defective' class of people that could not be elevated by education or social reform, as one had previously hoped. Redefining 'feeble-mindedness' as moral and biological deficiency, early twentieth-century eugenics thus classed this group as a 'lost race' without the capacity to advance to civilization.[31]

This attitude had a devastating impact on the schools and institutions supposed to serve those with intellectual disabilities. Driven by financial restrictions and eugenic motivations, they increasingly moved away from their educational mission to more cost-efficient custodial care and behavioural training. Moreover, together with sterilization, institutionalization became a prime eugenic instrument for controlling the 'feeble-minded'. As Allison Carey succinctly put it, 'most medical institutions operated as a form of social control and physical segregation in which inmates experienced neglect, abuse, and social, and civil "death"'.[32] Vice versa, other schools – including those for the deaf – increasingly tried to detect, and then rid themselves of, 'feeble-minded' students, who they considered lost to pedagogical efforts, and harmful to maintaining the image of successful deaf education.[33] Schools for the deaf felt the need to emphasize that they were regular schools, not to be mistaken with the asylums serving those lost to educational uplift. 'Admission into schools for the deaf has become more and more like that in the regular schools', sociologist Harry Best thus explained in 1914. They generally 'are open ... only to those able and fitted to be educated, and the mentally and physically disqualified are often rejected'.[34]

The eugenic impulse to stratify society – and school children – by their mental and physical traits went hand in hand with the progressive goal of creating more efficient schools. Engaging with questions of heredity, health, prevention, and efficiency, schools for the deaf were part of a larger process of normalizing and standardizing education, childhood, and disability. The abovementioned report on *Standardization, Efficiency, Heredity* proudly flashed the key words of this new scientific age. It announced a new 'epoch in the history of the education of the deaf'; the first attempt to measure 'along scientific lines' the quality and efficiency of deaf schools and the 'mental status' of their students. The goal of such modernization, guided only by 'utilitarian facts', was to discard 'old theories, customs, and traditions' in favour of new, scientifically proven paradigms that would make schools for the deaf more efficient.[35]

In the early decades of the twentieth century, schools thus became a testing ground for a number of social and scientific interventions in the name of progress. This was doubly true in special education. Here, the contemporary fascination with the otherness of people with disabilities met with the hopes put into the child as a developing being. Here, too, the relationship between the gospel of progress and efficiency, and of blaming the individual for deviance from the norm, became particularly evident. Many disciplines were involved in this process of norm-finding, efficiency, and exclusion. Child studies emerged as a field of its own, as psychologists, scientists, and educators mapped children's physical and intellectual development in relation to adults, their environment, and the larger evolutionary scale. It promised the application of modern science at home and in school. School hygiene, too, was part of this mission for progress through scientific reform. It was part of larger public health campaigns to improve hygienic conditions and to prevent and control infectious disease, but also congenital and hereditary conditions.[36]

At schools for the deaf, detecting, classifying, treating, and preventing hearing loss was an important part of this combination of educational, progressive, and eugenic motives. In a 1907 article in the *Volta Review* (the journal of the A. G. Bell Association) for example, the widely respected English deafness expert James Love Kerr argued that the early detection of hearing loss would not only improve medical treatment but also improve educational placement. Establishing a system of 'examination and supervision', he believed, would reduce the incidence of acquired hearing loss so drastically that in the future 'hardly any but the congenitally deaf will ask admission to our institutions'.[37] Discussing, in 1913, the causes of deafness, superintendent of the Utah School for the Deaf and Blind Frank Driggs similarly remarked on the 'necessity of a more careful study of children'. In particular, he hoped for a closer study of the 'exceptional child'. For Driggs this was not primarily a question of psychology or pedagogics, but of a detailed study of the causes of deafness, both hereditary and environmental. He was hopeful that this would mark the beginning of an era in which the 'breeding of more perfect human beings' would be possible. To achieve this goal, it was necessary to achieve a 'better cooperation between the doctor and the teacher in the study of children', yet also to consider restricting marriages between families carrying the same 'defective strain'.[38]

The Coolidge Fund for the Deaf: progressive science and promises of normalization

In its self-portrayal and mission, the Clarke School was very much part of these debates on studying, preventing, and overcoming disability and defect through modern, progressive methods. It was A. G. Bell who suggested that the school should have a research department of its own. In his position as president of the school board, he called, in 1921, for enlarging the school's endowment in order to improve buildings and to adjust infrastructure and scholarships. This had become necessary to serve the growing student population – by the mid-1920s, on average about 150 students, aged five to fifteen, attended the Clarke School. Yet Bell's plans went beyond mere investments in staff and infrastructure. Hoping to 'broaden [the school's] scope', he envisioned a future research department that would – like his own work – integrate science and education to tackle the problem of deafness.[39]

Bell did not live to see his vision realized; he died in 1922. Yet once again, the school could mobilize well-known figures to help them raise money for their ambitious plans. The President and First Lady, Calvin and Grace Goodhue Coolidge, in particular, drew attention to the Clarke School and America's deaf. They had met in Northampton where, before her marriage,

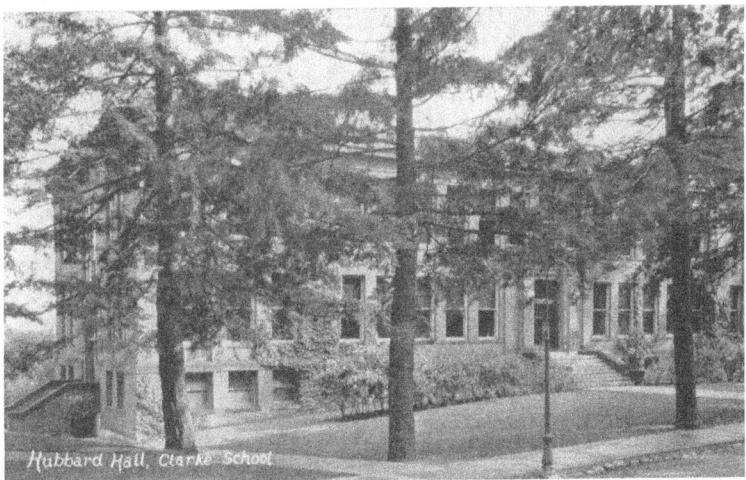

Figure 1 Postcard of Hubbard Hall, Clarke School For the Deaf, c. 1920s (reprinted with kind permission of the Department of Special Collections and University Archives, W. E. B. Du Bois Library, University of Massachusetts Amherst)

Grace Goodhue had worked at the Clarke School. As a 'young teacher endowed with rare gifts of tact, graciousness and sympathy', she had given 'herself wholly to the work of guiding little children across the narrow, perilous bridge which leads the deaf to the Promised Land of normal fellowship with their kind'.[40] The couple remained lifelong supporters of the school.

'Coolidge deaf fund launched', a November 1927 article in the *Pittsburgh Press* announced, and explained that at a luncheon 'plans for raising the endowment were outlined to many friends of the Coolidges'.[41] The eventual list of donors included 150 names, most of them contributing a sum between $500 and $5,000. Among the wealthier donors were Andrew Mellon, and the founders of the Woolworth Company Fred M. Kirby and Earle P. Charlton, who gave $100,000 each.[42] In a November 1928 letter to Charlton, Coolidge expressed his thanks and the hope that the fund 'may also help to arouse a greater interest in the problems of the deaf and in this humanitarian work which has seemingly failed to keep pace with progress in other fields'.[43]

As so often with charity, the Coolidge Fund's appeal was based more on the self-fashioning of the donors than on the lived realities of the recipients. Oralism, with its promise of progress and normalization, appealed to wealthy business people, from the founders of the Clarke School to the donors of the Coolidge Fund. It played a central role in presenting the deaf as a population able and willing to overcome adversity through hard work and the miracles of modern science. In a time in which, increasingly, people with disabilities were seen as 'defectives' unworthy of social reform, deaf children were singled out as innocent beings worthy of charity. Pointing to the uplifting powers of science, the Clarke School engaged in what historian Theresa Richardson called scientific charity. In preferring some causes to others, Richardson argued, philanthropists played an important role in legitimating and disseminating 'a medical paradigm in the name of human progress'. This pattern was particularly pervasive when it came to disability.[44]

The Coolidge Fund was accompanied by two publications appealing to the cause of transforming deaf lives via the educational-scientific uplift of oralism: *A Child at the Clarke School for the Deaf* (1927) and *The Coolidge Fund for the Clarke School and the Deaf* (1929). Garnering sympathy with its description of deaf children's normalcy, *A Child at the Clarke School for the Deaf* introduced its readers to the school's 'healthy, normal looking' students, 'bright-eyed' and 'expectant' of their lessons. Throughout its thirty pages, the booklet contrasted the situation of the 'lonely deaf child, frustrated, "walled in," emotionally at sea' with the humanizing and liberating impact of oralist education, as the 'the way out into the sunlight where normal people talk and laugh and weep together'. The school left no doubt that the deaf child was indeed 'normal', merely an 'exiled spirit' to whom speech gave back their very 'own birthright'.[45]

Deaf children, the school insisted, 'must not be institutionalized nor segregated'. In a time when the segregation and institutionalization of disabled people seemed like the solution for a host of social problems, the Clarke School went to great pains to make clear that for the deaf, residential schooling was only a temporary stage on their way to becoming 'responsible citizens' who 'in many cases make contributions of great value to the sum total of human achievement'. Such adamant assertions of their students' inherent normalcy were a defence both from old prejudice and new eugenic stigma.[46]

Yet this language of liberation also set up a clear hierarchy of knowledge and agency between helpless deaf people and the heroic oralist teachers who 'liberated these prisoners of silence'.[47] Unlike deaf teachers, who had often acted as role models introducing their students to signing and the larger deaf community, the hearing teachers at the Clarke School stood firmly on the side of hearing normalcy. Oralist education was presented as an uplifting parable of virtues and rewards, a satisfying moral tale about overcoming disability by hard work. As in virtually all disability narratives in early twentieth-century America, it was the individual who had to adapt and hide their differences in order to pass as 'normal'. Giving the deaf child the 'tools' for success, teachers demanded '[p]atience and eagerness and determination'. If 'he works', the booklet promised, 'he will learn to be more like other children' – a logic that implicitly associated 'oral failures', deaf people who did not pass as almost-hearing, with a lack of work ethics and determination.[48] Unspoken, yet always present in this unrealistic glorification of oralist success, was its negative counterpart, the scenario to be avoided at all cost: the deaf child who would grow up to associate with the deaf community, who would segregate themselves from hearing society, marry a deaf partner, and thus perpetuate deaf difference linguistically, culturally – and, perhaps, biologically. As A. G. Bell had explained in his *Memoir*, 'segregation really lies at the root of the whole matter' of deaf intermarriage. While the Clarke School could not (yet) fulfil Bell's ideal of co-educating deaf and hearing children, it followed the principle of maintaining a 'normal', that is, a hearing, 'environment during the period of education'. Casting sign language as an 'artificial barrier', teachers aimed to create an atmosphere in which oralism 'penetrates behind the child's mind'.[49]

Whereas *A Child at the Clarke School* focused predominantly on the school's educational work, the 1929 *The Coolidge Fund for the Clarke School and the Deaf* turned hearing loss into a much wider humanitarian concern. The booklet painted a dire picture of the situation of America's deaf people. It claimed that the problem of deafness in the United States was severely underestimated. The 1920 US census had counted roughly 53,000 deaf people. By including the hard-of-hearing and those with moderate hearing loss, the *Coolidge Fund* turned deafness into a problem affecting an estimated ten million people. These numbers pointed to the 'vital need for an organization which will meet and grapple with the problem of the deaf in America on a national scale'.[50] That there might be a lack of organizations serving the deaf was a peculiar claim, although convenient to fundraising rhetoric. By the early twentieth century, a host of local, regional, and national organizations represented the concerns of deaf people and teachers for the deaf, including the Volta Bureau (established by A. G. Bell in 1887 to promote oralism and research on deafness) and the highly active NAD.[51] It was true, however, that there was no school-based research unit that combined science and pedagogy. This was, the booklet claimed, because deafness had long been treated as 'an incurable affliction', and thus, 'we are today further behind in adequate practical dealing with the problem of deafness than with any other social problem'. Such wording rendered deafness as a social ill, a (potentially curable) disease at the scale of polio, tuberculosis, and other conditions deserving of large-scale public attention.[52]

The Clarence W. Barron Research Department: collaboration and friction in an oralist setting

By the end of the 1928–1929 school year, the fundraising for the Coolidge Fund was complete. It amounted to the impressive sum of two million dollars, of which 300,000 were dedicated to setting up the new research department with its subdivisions for psychology, heredity research, and experimental phonetics. It was named after the late financial journalist Clarence W. Barron, president of Dow Jones & Company, who had used his contacts and business skills to organize the fundraising.[53] In the annual report, the head of the school corporation, Henry D. Wild, once more pointed to the benefits of deafness research. He assured that the school would continue to function 'much as before', yet 'with even greater efficiency' now that 'special attention' was given to research. Since its foundation, he wrote, the Clarke School had proudly 'led in the building of new ways in the most difficult form of education known'. Conscious 'of its new opportunity and of its increasing responsibility', it now was pioneering again in an 'unexplored field' that held much promise.[54]

Even before the Coolidge Fund was completed, the school had begun looking for suitable researchers. Here, they capitalized on long-standing ties to neighbouring Smith College. In 1928, eminent Gestalt psychologist and newly appointed Smith College professor Kurt Koffka agreed to direct Clarke's psychology research, and began hiring co-workers and assistants. Research aimed to explore the emotional and intellectual differences between deaf and hearing children, with particular emphasis on their 'conscious thinking'.[55] In 1930, Koffka handed over his position to Austrian Gestalt psychologist Fritz Heider, who later became a founding figure of social psychology.[56] The position as head for the heredity division was filled in 1930 with young anthropologist Morris Steggerda, again through the connection with Smith.[57] Finally, in the 1932–1933 school year, the division for experimental phonetics began working under Clarence V. Hudgins. Studying the speech of deaf and hearing individuals, its goal was to 'eliminate some of the defects' in deaf people's speech, and thus to improve oralist education.[58] In later decades, Hudgins' division would also explore the use of assistive devices, such as hearing aids.

In these early years of the research department, a lasting pattern of division of work formed between the Clarke School and outside researchers, with important implications for how deafness was researched, and how research was applied. Both sides profited from their cooperation. For the school, employing outside researchers maximized their resources and provided access to academic research and networks. Moreover, it associated them with prestigious names and institutions. For outside researchers, the school provided access to an interesting research population, data, research assistants, and not least, the additional title of head of a research division. For Steggerda, Koffka, Heider, and others, who later worked with the school, this was a part-time obligation, usually next to a professorship or position elsewhere (often at Smith College). As supervising investigator, they were mainly responsible for devising theoretical frameworks, research plans, and directing analysis. For the more menial tasks of day-to-day research, the school recruited from their own pool of teachers. Alongside their other tasks, these teacher-researchers – who had much enthusiasm for, but little background in research – carried out observations and examinations, made records, and filed data.

Yet the collaboration between the Clarke School and these researchers also created moments of dissonance and disconnect about the meaning of deafness, the abilities of deaf people, and the goals of research. Certainly, both sides shared certain beliefs and assumptions. Most importantly, they agreed that deafness was a disease, pathology, or disability to be fixed, ameliorated, or prevented (although psychological research would come to question this). Yet even in the 1930s, what was to be fixed and how so depended on professional outlook, institutional context, and personal beliefs. For the Clarke School, all research operated under the unified goal of oralism: ameliorating the effects of deafness in their students, so that they could pass as quasi-hearing, and preventing its occurrence. All three fields of research – psychology, phonetics, and heredity research – were to contribute equally to this ideal. Thus, Henry Wild noted in 1930 that the study of psychology 'may well lead to discoveries from which much practical pedagogical value may be gained'. At the same time, he believed that the time might be 'ripe for addressing ourselves to the possible hygienic prevention of deafness through the study of hereditary processes'. In this field, the school 'may again seize an unusual opportunity in sponsoring progress'. Here, heredity research became part of ensuring the school's future success in achieving scientific progress and social amelioration. 'For us', Wild concluded, 'the chief thing is that the psychological, as well as the biological, study of deafness must inevitably lead to practical classroom benefits'.[59]

Outside researchers, on the other hand, were not obligated to, or even familiar with, oralist ideals. Especially with psychology and heredity research, they were not usually experts on deafness (nor had they worked with deaf people before), but were hired for their general expertise in their field. At home in the world of academic science, their interests and goals of research usually differed, too. Whereas school staff was invested in its holistic vision of science as a means of forming deaf children into productive citizens and full human beings, they saw deafness as an abstract phenomenon. And rather than taking on the teacher's role as a paternalistic guiding figure, they approached deaf students with the distanced gaze of the scientist appraising an interesting population that could enlighten larger theoretical questions. This did not necessarily result in less pathologizing, medicalizing, or paternalistic perspectives. In heredity research, the next chapter will show, eugenicists and educators formed an alliance over the shared goal of preventing hereditary deafness, and the apparent truism that it was best if deaf people did not marry each other. Yet, as this chapter and the next show, such an alliance did not mean that different groups of professionals agreed about the best way to achieve this goal, and the reproductive agency that should be granted to deaf people. Oralism fostered in educators a paternalistic (and often equally intrusive) sense of responsibility for deaf people, coupled with a strong belief in their normalcy. Other professionals and the general public often harboured more negative preconceptions, especially in a time that tended to equate all disability with defectiveness and degeneration.

The work of Clarke's psychology division shows, however, that an abstract distance could also help foster a more relativistic and less pathologizing perspective. The research conducted in the 1930s and 1940s, by the head of the division Fritz Heider and his wife and co-worker Grace Moore Heider, was guided by Gestalt and social psychology, and by the fact that they remained outsiders to the school's closed-off pedagogical and social world. Indeed, falling in love immediately upon Heider's arrival in Northampton in August

1930, and soon planning their marriage, they found that the school considered such a union inappropriate and even threatened to fire Heider. Heider and Moore, on the other hand, considered such a puritan, small-town intrusion into their private lives inappropriate, and were married by the end of the year. Fritz Heider's first impression of the school was of the strict order and discipline in which students were held, which to him seemed to go against the nature of children.[60] He also noted that teachers did not take students 'as a human being on the same level', did not 'take them serious', and treated them in a condescending manner that interrupted their natural learning process.[61]

As Gestalt psychologists, the Heiders were interested in the relationship between perception, thought, and language; as social psychologists, they were interested in the relationship between individual and society. For both interests, deaf students provided interesting insights – just because they were different. Tasked by the school with a study of speech and lip-reading skills, the psychologists concluded that deaf children could and should not be expected to pronounce words in the same manner as the hearing – the very goal of oralist education – because their phenomenological and sensory experience was different. Within contemporary deaf and special education, this was a highly unusual, even revolutionary conclusion. The Heiders also conducted a survey of deaf adults, including Clarke School alumni, trying to capture their lived reality and attitudes towards deafness. They observed that after graduating, many deaf adults predominantly lived in signing deaf communities that minimized contact with the hearing. This was a well-known fact, yet one that professionals usually ignored or judged as oralist failure. To the psychologists, however, who were not obliged to the oralist goal of making deaf children pass as almost-hearing, it was perfectly reasonable that deaf people lived in a different phenomenological and social sphere. Deafness, they concluded, was a relational condition, and the deaf a 'social minority' whose problems were caused at least as much by 'the attitudes of the hearing than by the sense defect itself'.[62]

It is an ironic twist of history that it was here, at the country's leading oralist school, that psychologists first produced a sociological study of deafness as a relational, interpersonal phenomenon and of deaf people as a social minority – long before such definitions became fashionable in linguistics or social science. These results are telling for the relative freedom the school allowed the scientists they hired to conduct research, yet also for how the school incorporated – or didn't incorporate – results into their educational practice. For the school, psychological research was a means towards their overall goal of transforming deaf children into successful citizens able to pass as 'normal' in hearing society. Results that did not align with this worldview were ignored.

Conclusion

Much like today, schools in early twentieth-century America were important locations of social and scientific reform, places to produce healthier, better, and more productive citizens. Special education, in particular, engaged with this vision. It took part, simultaneously, in moulding the careless child into a responsible adult, and in transforming the 'defective' or 'subnormal' student into a productive citizen. Complementing its educational programme with a multi-disciplinary research department, the Clarke School embraced both strands. With its research, it took part in the ongoing medicalization and standardization of childhood, education, and disability. Far more than just speech-training and education, the school provided, in the words of historian Stephen Petrina, an 'educational hygiene' that was to become engrained in a student's very being. By the early twentieth century, Petrina writes, schools 'had become an educational dispensary of "therapeutic milieu"' that imagined students as patients to be improved.[63] With the creation of the research department, students thus quite literally also became objects of research, subjected to audiological tests, health exams, and genealogical investigations.

Certainly, oralism embodied such a therapeutic vision, yet it also aimed to transcend it. Fears of the deaf child left behind, isolated without real language, drove the urgency with which the Clarke School pushed for salvation through oralism. Deafness was less an innate difference – oralism promised normalcy and assimilation – than an (evolutionary) stage to be overcome. Emphasizing deaf people's inherent normalcy turned deafness into something to be shed and left behind, either – in the current generation – by learning speech and inconspicuous behaviour, or – in the next – by breeding out the 'defective' trait.

Heredity research at the Clarke School was embedded in this framework concerned with the inheritance of defect, but also with the standardization and efficiency of education, with mental and social hygiene, evolutionary thought, and childhood studies. Like most of its contemporaries, the school embraced eugenics as a new and promising instrument of social change that combined measures of public health and education, and, like other branches of science, could contribute to the betterment of humankind and society. Embracing eugenics as a means of betterment while rejecting for deaf people the label of 'defectives' makes once again visible how closely eugenic policies were tied to ableist notions of productive citizenship, social usefulness, and bourgeois morality.

When looking at research at the Clarke School, it is important to note that its self-portrayal as a place of scientific progress and uplift was carefully curated, and that this image was at least as important as any real effect of research on teaching and daily operations. In this, the school certainly was not alone, yet looking behind the scenes brings out fissures and dissonances in the familiar story of science and progress. Such a perspective also complicates narratives that have portrayed research of disability and deafness during the first half of the century as a uniform process of medicalization and professionalization.

In a time that strongly believed in 'fixing' and overcoming disability via science and hard work, oralism had a tremendous appeal. Not everyone, however, was committed to or familiar with its holistic ideal of transformation and normalization. The very set-up of Clarke's research department brought to the school researchers who were interested in deafness for different reasons, and interacted with deaf people in different ways. To these outside scientists, deaf students were primarily an interesting research population among which certain hereditary or psychological traits could be studied. Certainly, the first decades of the twentieth century were predominantly a time in which different disciplines medicalized and pathologized deafness, and, in doing so, excluded deaf people's perspectives and limited their agency.

Yet psychological research under Fritz and Grace Moore Heider makes visible that even within this generally medicalizing framework we can discover the germs for later, more diverse (and less pathologizing) perceptions of deafness and deaf people. At the Clarke School, psychological and heredity research moved on completely separate paths, yet these new psychosocial approaches would influence genetic research and counselling in the 1950s. The relationship between the school and its psychologists also shows that the pragmatic collaboration between Clarke and its researchers could produce results that went against the grain of oralist beliefs. In the school's closed-off and self-perpetuating world, such non-fitting elements were usually ignored. As becomes clear in the next chapter on the work of the heredity division, such interdisciplinary alliances between school and outside experts were often temporary and shifted with new insights, changing institutional context, or professional orientations. What hereditary deafness meant, and how deaf people should be counselled, depended much on whether one was an oralist teacher, anthropologist, or medical geneticist.

Notes

1 Parts of this chapter appeared in M. A. Schmidt, 'Extremely concerned and puzzled: hereditary deafness research at Clarke School for the Deaf, 1930–1983', in B. H. Greenwald and J. J. Murray (eds), *In Our Own Hands: Essays in Deaf History, 1780–1970* (Washington, DC: Gallaudet University Press, 2016), pp. 193–209;

M. A. Schmidt, 'Planes of phenomenological experience: the psychology of deafness as an early example of American Gestalt psychology, 1928–1940', *History of Psychology*, 20:4 (2017), 347–64. See also Clarke School for the Deaf, *The Coolidge Fund for the Clarke School and the Deaf* (New York: Coolidge Fund, 1929).

2 Douglas Baynton has analysed most extensively the impact of evolutionary thought, social Darwinism, nativism, and capitalism on perceptions of deafness, disability, and sign language. See in particular Baynton, *Forbidden Signs* and '"These pushful days"'. For the overlap between eugenics, social reform, and the perception of individuals with a disability as socially and morally defiant see e.g. A. C. Carey, *On the Margins of Citizenship: Intellectual Disability and Civil Rights in Twentieth-Century America* (Philadelphia, PA: Temple University Press, 2010), pp. 53–71; Kline, *Better Race*, pp. 7–31.

3 This strict division between a German oral and a French manual method is to some extent a retrospective construction that does not do justice to the variety of methods used in eighteenth- and nineteenth-century Europe. See e.g. the contribution to M. Schmidt and A. Werner (eds), *Zwischen Fremdbestimmung und Autonomie: Neue Impulse zur Gehörlosengeschichte in Deutschland, Österreich und der Schweiz* (Bielefeld: transcript, 2019).

4 See Baynton, *Forbidden Signs*, pp. 15–35; Edwards, *Words*, pp. 33–49.

5 For the role of residential schools and the development of the deaf community see Van Cleve and Crouch, *Place*, pp. 29, 47, 87–93; Edwards, *Words*, pp. 51–114.

6 For Hubbard's advocacy see Edwards, *Words*, pp. 143–59.

7 Baynton, *Forbidden Signs*, pp. 9, 139–45. For similarities between the histories of deaf people, African Americans and other minorities, difference and passing as normal also see C. Krentz, *Writing Deafness: the Hearing Line in Nineteenth-century American Literature*. (Chapel Hill, NC: University of North Carolina Press, 2007). For the impact of evolutionary thought on understanding childhood see S. Shuttleworth, *The Mind of the Child: Child Development in Literature, Science, and Medicine, 1840–1900* (Oxford: Oxford University Press, 2010), pp. 5–8, 237–64.

8 See M. E. Numbers, *My Words Fell on Deaf Ears: An Account of the First Hundred Years of the Clarke School for the Deaf* (Washington, DC: Alexander Graham Bell Association for the Deaf, 1974), pp. 17–19.

9 Clarke School for the Deaf, *A Child at the Clarke School for the Deaf* (Northampton, MA: Clarke School for the Deaf, 1927), p. 28.

10 L. Schlesinger, 'The methods controversy in American deaf education: a sociological perspective' (Honor thesis, Smith College, 1977), 137.

11 See e.g. Van Cleve and Crouch, *Place*, p. 148. For a nuanced analysis of Bell's position on deafness and eugenics see Greenwald, 'Alexander Graham Bell'.

12 For Bell's life and role at the Clarke School see Greenwald, 'Alexander Graham Bell', pp. 57–69; C. D. Mackenzie, *Alexander Graham Bell, the Man Who Contracted Space* (Boston, MA: Houghton Mifflin Company, 1928), pp. 54–6; Numbers, *My Words Fell on Deaf Ears*, pp. 73–4.

13 For a history of deafness and deaf people on Martha's Vineyard see N. E. Groce, *Everyone Here Spoke Sign Language: Hereditary Deafness on Martha's Vineyard* (Cambridge, MA: Harvard University Press, 1987).
14 Bell, *Memoir*, pp. 4, 41.
15 *Ibid.*, p. 47.
16 *Ibid.*, p. 42.
17 *Ibid.*, pp. 4, 46. Greenwald, 'Alexander Graham Bell', pp. 15, 50, 80, 91.
18 Greenwald, 'Alexander Graham Bell', pp. 13, 72–4 159–60. For the history of the ABA and its Eugenics Committee see B. A. Kimmelman, 'The American Breeders' Association: genetics and eugenics in an agricultural context, 1903–13', *Social Studies of Science*, 13:2 (1983), 163–204.
19 Greenwald, 'Alexander Graham Bell', pp. 171–200. For Bell's later position on eugenics see A. G. Bell, *A Few Thoughts Concerning Eugenics* (Washington, DC: Judd & Detweiler, 1908).
20 Apart from the works on eugenics already mentioned, for more on the confluence between eugenics and progressive thought see, in particular, M. Freeden, 'Eugenics and progressive thought: a study in ideological affinity', *Historical Journal*, 22 (1979), 645–71.
21 Carey, *On the Margins of Citizenship*, p. 53.
22 For perceptions of 'feeble-mindedness' see e.g. Kline, *Better Race*, pp. 7–94; Carey, *On the Margins of Citizenship*, pp. 52–81. For the development of sterilization legislation see P. Reilly, *The Surgical Solution: A History of Involuntary Sterilization in the United States* (Baltimore, MD: Johns Hopkins University Press, 1991); Schoen, *Choice & Coercion*; I. R. Dowbiggin, *The Sterilization Movement and Global Fertility in the Twentieth Century* (New York: Oxford University Press, 2008).
23 See A. M. Tuchman, 'Diabetes and "defective" genes in the twentieth-century United States', *Journal of the History of Medicine and Allied Sciences*, 70:1 (2013), 1–33.
24 Burch gives the fullest account of right restrictions during the progressive and eugenic era. See S. Burch, *Signs of Resistance: American Deaf Cultural History, 1900 to World War II* (New York: New York University Press, 2002), pp. 129–67. How many deaf people were actually sterilized has not been well documented. Lane, Hoffmeister and Bahan write, without reference to specific sources, that eugenics' 'well-publicized pursuits led untold numbers of Deaf people to abandon plans for marriage and reproduction or to submit to voluntary sterilization, and untold numbers of hearing parents to have their Deaf children sterilized'. See Lane et al., *Journey*, p. 381.
25 See 'NAD history' under www.nad.org/about-us/nad-history/#1970s [accessed 30 May 2019].
26 Robinson, O., '"We are a different class": ableist rhetoric in deaf America 1880–1920', in S. Burch and A. Kafer (eds), *Deaf and Disability Studies: Interdisciplinary Perspectives* (Washington, DC: Gallaudet University Press, 2010), pp. 5–21, here p. 7.

27 See Burch, *Signs of Resistance*, pp. 149–52; Robinson, '"We are a different class"'.
28 Burch, *Signs of Resistance*, p. 142.
29 Burch, *Signs of Resistance*, pp. 4, 136, 144, 170; Robinson, '"We are a different class"', pp. 14–15. Also see William Ennis' analysis of the discussion of eugenics and deaf intermarriage among Gallaudet faculty and students. Ennis, 'Hereditarian ideas', pp. 42–125.
30 R. O. Johnson, *Standardization, Efficiency, Heredity: Schools for the Deaf* (Indianapolis, IN: Burford, 1920), pp. 58, 60, 101, 208, 15.
31 H. H. Goddard, *The Kallikak Family: A Study in the Heredity of Feeble-Mindedness* (New York: The Macmillan Company, 1912). For Goddard see L. Zenderland, *Measuring Minds: Henry Herbert Goddard and the Origins of American Intelligence Testing* (Cambridge: Cambridge University Press, 1998). Smith and Wehmeyer have traced the story of Deborah Kallikak – whose real name was Emma Wolverton – and how she came to be a showcase of eugenic degeneration. See D. J. Smith and M. L. Wehmeyer, 'Who was Deborah Kallikak?', *Intellectual and Developmental Disabilities*, 50:2 (2012), 169–78.
32 Carey, *On the Margins of Citizenship*, pp. 13, 146.
33 For this development see R. L. Osgood, *The History of Special Education: A Struggle for Equality in American Public Schools* (Westport, CT: Praeger, 2008), pp. 34–6; R. L. Osgood, 'Education in the name of "improvement": the influence of eugenic thought and practice in Indiana's public schools, 1900–1930', *Indiana Magazine of History*, 106:3 (2010), 272–99.
34 H. Best, *The Deaf: Their Position in Society and the Provision for their Education in the United States*. (New York: T. Y. Crowell Co., 1914), p. 252.
35 Johnson, *Standardization*, pp. 19, 23, 26. For progressive thought and the medicalization of education see e.g. S. Petrina, 'The medicalization of education: a historiographic synthesis', *History of Education Quarterly*, 46:4 (2007), 503–31; W. J. Reese, *Power and the Promise of School Reform: Grassroots Movements during the Progressive Era* (Boston, MA: Routledge & Kegan Paul, 1986); R. E. Callahan, *Education and the Cult of Efficiency: A Study of the Social Forces that Have Shaped the Administration of the Public Schools* (Chicago, IL: University of Chicago Press, 1962).
36 See e.g. R. A. Meckel, *Classrooms and Clinics: Urban Schools and the Protection and Promotion of Child Health, 1870–1930* (New Brunswick, NJ: Rutgers University Press, 2013). For the development of child studies in particular see e.g. Shuttleworth, *Mind*.
37 J. K. Love, 'The study of the deaf child', *Volta Review*, 9 (1907), 449–64, here 449.
38 F. Driggs, 'The causes of deafness', *Volta Review*, 15 (1913), 330–4, here 330, 333.
39 Bell, A. G., 'Report of the corporation', *Fifty-Fourth Annual Report of the Clarke School for the Deaf. Northampton, Mass. For the Year Ending August 31, 1921*, 7–10, here 7. In the following abbreviated as *Clarke School Annual Report*. The student numbers are taken from the 1927 report, see *Clarke School Annual Report*, 60 (1927), 12.

40 Clarke School, *Coolidge Fund*, pp. 9, 11.
41 R. Tucker, 'Coolidge Deaf Fund launched: school where Grace Goodhue taught is beneficiary', *Pittsburgh Press* (16 November 1928).
42 List of donors, insert in copy of Clarke School, *A Child at the Clarke School* at the New York Historical Society library.
43 Letter from Calvin Coolidge to Mr. Earle P. Charlton regarding the Coolidge Fund, 14 November 1928, insert in copy of Clarke School, *A Child at the Clarke School* at the New York Historical Society library.
44 T. R. Richardson, *The Century of the Child: The Mental Hygiene Movement and Social Policy in the United States and Canada* (Albany, NY: State University of New York Press, 1989), p. 27. For the rhetoric of disability and charity in particular see S. C. Moeschen, 'Suffering silences, woeful afflictions: physical disability, melodrama, and the American Charity movement', *Comparative Drama*, 40:4 (2011), 433–54.
45 Clarke School, *A Child at the Clarke School*, pp. 3, 5, 8, 18. 25. For the widespread portrayal of deafness as isolation and exclusion see D. C. Baynton, '"A silent exile on this earth": the metaphorical construction of deafness in the 19th century', *American Quarterly*, 44 (1992), 216–43.
46 Clarke School, *A Child at the Clarke School*, pp. 9, 21.
47 *Ibid.*, p. 27.
48 *Ibid.*, pp. 18–19.
49 Bell, *Memoir*, p. 45; Clarke School, *A Child at the Clarke School*, pp. 9–10.
50 Clarke School, *Coolidge Fund*, p. 17. For US Census numbers on deafness see Best, *The Deaf*, p. 5; H. Best, *The Deaf-Mute Population of the United States, 1920: A Statistical Analysis of the Data Obtained at the Fourteenth Decentennial Census* (Washington, DC: U.S. Government Printing Office, 1928).
51 See Greenwald, 'Alexander Graham Bell', pp. 23, 66; Van Cleve and Crouch, *Place*, p. 93.
52 Clarke School, *Coolidge Fund*, p. 18. While there was no other school-based research organization, in 1923 the Johns Hopkins University founded an Otological Research Laboratory under S. J. Crowe that mainly focused on environmental causes. See S. J. Crowe and J. W. Baylor, 'The prevention of deafness', *Journal of the American Medical Association*, 112:7 (1939), 585–90.
53 See Clarke School, *Coolidge Fund*, p. 48. For the role of Barron see C. A. Yale, *Years of Building: Memories of a Pioneer in a Special Field of Education* (New York: L. MacVeagh, The Dial Press, 1931), p. 293.
54 H. D. Wild, 'Report of the corporation', *Clarke School Annual Report*, 62 (1929), 11–15, here 12–13.
55 M. Eberhardt, 'Report of the research department', *Clarke School Annual Report*, 62 (1929), 25. Also see I. F. Wood, 'Report of the corporation', *Clarke School Annual Report*, 61 (1928), 11–14.
56 H. D. Wild, 'Report of the corporation', *Clarke School Annual Report*, 63 (1930), 11–13.

57 B. N. Leonard, 'Report of the principal', *Clarke School Annual Report*, 63 (1930), 17–22.
58 'Report, division of experimental phonetics', *Clarke School Annual Report*, 61 (1933), 31–5.
59 Wild, 'Report of the corporation', 13–14.
60 See F. Heider, *The Life of a Psychologist: An Autobiography* (Lawrence, KS: University Press of Kansas, 1983), pp. 87–97, 128–9.
61 In the German original: 'Das Kind wird nicht genommen als Mensch auf gleichem Niveau, nicht ernst genommen', University Archives, Kenneth Spencer Research Library, University of Kansas, Personal papers of Fritz Heider, 'First impressions of Clarke School', Fritz Heider collection, PP. 343, Box 26, Folder 25.
62 F. Heider and G. M. Heider, *Studies in the Psychology of the Deaf, No. 2.* (Evanston, IL: American Psychological Association, 1941), p. 120. For the Clarke School psychology research and the Heiders' work see Schmidt, 'Planes of phenomenological experience'.
63 Petrina, 'The medicalization of education', 508, 527.

2

CONCERNED AND PUZZLED: HEREDITY RESEARCH AND COUNSELLING AT THE CLARKE SCHOOL, 1930–1960

Under the guidance of anthropologist Morris Steggerda, the Clarke School's heredity research division took up work in the 1929–1930 school year. Already a leader in oral education, the school now aimed to establish itself in heredity research, too. This was not an easy task in a place where the staff was knowledgeable about education and phonetics, yet had neither basic science training nor research experience. However, collaborating with leading researchers and institutions, Clarke managed to put together one of the most extensive longitudinal databases on the inheritance of deafness worldwide.

Covering the period from the 1930s to the 1960s, the school's heredity research fell into a time of immense changes in eugenics, genetics, and genetic counselling. During this time, the coercive, state-driven, and biased eugenics of the 1920s, 1930s, and 1940s grew into the modern medical genetics of the 1950s and 1960s, which, increasingly, emphasized individual autonomy. Historians have given much attention to the fraught, ritualized, and incomplete manner in which geneticists, physicians, biologists, or anthropologists revoked their eugenic past, and have pointed to the continuities of eugenic thought in gender and family roles, in the post-war celebration of the middle-class family, or in the continuing restriction of reproductive rights of people of colour or with disabilities.[1] Some have argued that the shift from coercive methods to more moderate and less restrictive genetic counselling was engendered by a more sophisticated understanding of hereditary mechanisms.[2] Yet such changing beliefs about reproductive autonomy were more complicated than a simple progress from ignorance and bias to knowledge and true science.

In deafness research, too, we can see such changes. When Clarke's heredity division began working in the 1930s, oralist educators and heredity researchers shared a basic goal: it was crucial to identify individuals whose deafness was inherited and to discourage them from marrying another such person.

Moreover, given that one could not clearly distinguish hereditary from other forms of deafness, it was best that deaf people did not marry each other at all. By the 1950s and 1960s, however, with geneticists capable of making more precise predictions about whether or not a deaf couple would have deaf children, this consensus would begin to unravel. What was to be prevented, and how so, was no longer quite so clear. Was it deaf intermarriage per se, or merely deaf offspring? And whose decision was this, anyway, that of professionals, or of the couple and family involved? Increasingly, geneticists and educators would come to disagree.

The Clarke School provides rare insight to an institution in which a eugenic programme remained almost unchanged for decades, at some point progressive, yet increasingly out of touch with larger developments. The school's educators and officials were not invested in – and sometimes not even aware of – the (often superficial) attempts to sanitize genetics from its now unwanted eugenic past. Although the school collaborated with leading actors in eugenics and medical genetics, they developed their own culture and paradigm of heredity research and its application. It was deeply embedded in the oralist mission to normalize students and assimilate them into hearing society. Education, medicine, and eugenics intertwined in the mission to turn deaf children into 'normal', productive, and responsible citizens – responsible, too, when it came to choosing the 'right' – that is, a hearing – spouse.

Placing the Clarke School in a network of interdisciplinary and international research, this chapter will follow its changing role alongside three different axes: advances in understanding genetic deafness; the professions and interdisciplinary alliances that drove these advances; and continuity and change in beliefs of how to best address genetic conditions and counsel those affected. Placing the school in this larger framework makes visible different eugenic traditions and different beliefs about the nature of deafness, which could increase fears about the uncontrolled reproduction of so-called 'defectives' or engender the more individualized genetic counselling with which we are familiar today.

Tracing an elusive trait: early twentieth-century hereditary deafness research

The Clarke School was not the only place interested in the inheritance of deafness. For early twentieth-century teachers of the deaf, it became increasingly important to know why and when their students had lost their hearing. They considered this an important issue for educational placement and administration, and for improving public health by identifying and preventing certain forms of hearing loss – or at least learning more about when and where they occurred. Professionals distinguished broadly between two categories: adventitious or acquired deafness (through disease or accident), and hereditary or congenital deafness. In many cases, however, it was difficult, if not impossible to determine when and why a child had become deaf. Sometimes, the onset of deafness could be clearly associated with accidents, injuries, or infectious diseases such as meningitis, scarlet fever, and ear infections. Often, however, there was no such direct correlation. In such cases, congenital deafness served as a broad category for both hereditary cases and hearing loss acquired in utero. However, in a time before new-born hearing tests, when deafness was often noted only when toddlers did not react to noise or start speaking, it could be difficult to draw the line between congenital and acquired deafness. In the 1910s and 1920s, careful estimates classed between 20 to 30 per cent of cases as hereditary or congenital.[3]

Professionals were aware that congenital and hereditary deafness were 'not altogether one and the same thing', as sociologist Harry Best put it in his 1914 survey of the American deaf population.[4] Yet how to distinguish hereditary and congenital cases, and how, exactly, deafness was passed on from generation to generation were far from clear. In the wake of Bell's 1884 *Memoir*, scientists, educators, and deaf people themselves had been trying to find patterns of inheritance in order to prove or disprove his theory about the dangers of creating a deaf race. Gallaudet professor Edward Allen Fay, who was supportive of sign language and a fluent signer himself, provided the most exhaustive study. His 1898 *Marriages of the Deaf in America* compiled several thousand questionnaires into a data set still used in modern genetics. Fay went further than Bell, who had only studied deaf couples and their children, and also looked at the pattern in which deafness occurred in their wider families. He concluded that in regard to passing on deafness it was 'exceedingly dangerous for a deaf person to marry a blood relative'.[5] This – and here Fay differed from Bell – seemed to be independent from whether the partner was hearing or deaf. These results were puzzling, and Fay was not sure what conclusions to draw.[6]

In the 1880s, Bell, Fay, and other early researchers looked at heredity with a pre-Mendelian understanding. By the 1910s, Mendelism had become the guiding paradigm of heredity research. It gave scientists an explanatory model to study and predict a wide range of mental, physical, and moral traits. However, proving that any such traits were passed on as single recessive or dominant units was difficult, if not impossible, especially in more complex phenomena. Nevertheless, Mendelian genetics remained highly appealing, not least because it supported the belief in the ability to predict and direct heredity.[7] Deafness research was a good example for both this belief, and for the difficulties of applying simple Mendelian patterns to a highly complex phenomenon that decades later turned out to be determined by a myriad of different genes.

In the 1920s and 1930s, scientists believed deafness to be caused by one or a few single genes. A recessive pattern of inheritance seemed likely, given that, often, two deaf people had hearing as well as deaf children. Comparing pedigrees from different families, however, provided as much confusion as confirmation for these theories. Faced with these analytic difficulties, professionals often resorted to older metaphors. A 1912 *Volta Review* article on 'Heredity and intermarriage', for example, simply stated that the 'fatal tendency of deafness lurks in the family line'.[8]

One of the most sophisticated analyses arguing for recessive inheritance was William J. Tinkle's 1932 doctoral dissertation 'Deafness as a eugenical problem'.[9] Tinkle, then a University of Ohio student of zoology, had gone through the records of the Ohio State and Columbus Schools for the Deaf and had found thirty-one families in which two deaf parents had sent at least one of their children there. Deafness, he wrote, 'runs in families just like traits known to be hereditary, causing children to resemble parents closely'. Previous research, he noted, had supposed that deafness was a recessive trait. Yet was there only one single gene? If this was true, all children born to two deaf parents should be deaf, too. Since this was not the case – in Tinkle's Ohio population it was only 70 per cent – there must be at least two recessive genes involved. He suggested that one form might cause hearing loss for high tones, the other for low tones, though he could not prove this theory. Yet no matter the exact pattern of inheritance, he believed it was necessary to 'promote marriages between deaf and hearing persons, which are desirable if the deaf marry at all'. Following Bell, he advised to 'stop segregating the deaf' and to 'increase our day schools, teach lip reading and oral speech, and thus avoid taking deaf persons out of their normal environment'.[10]

For Tinkle and other early twentieth-century researchers, the very fact that hereditary deafness could not be clearly defined made it an even more pressing eugenic problem. For them, deaf intermarriage was a question of education as much as of public health, of changing deaf people's social environment as a means of changing their hereditary constitution. For the Clarke School, too, the fact that hereditary deafness could not be clearly grasped and controlled made it even more threatening. Unlike other researchers and institutions, however, Clarke had the resources to research it over a long period of time and with a large research population – and to apply research to this very population. It also had a wider scope of analysis.

Heredity research at an oralist school: audiograms and pedigrees

Clarke's heredity research was shaped by different influences: the school's oralist paradigm, its focus on the audiological measurement of hearing loss, and the knowledge and approaches brought in by outside scientists. The first to leave his mark was anthropologist Morris Steggerda. Born in Michigan in 1900 to immigrants from the Netherlands, he had received an MA in 1923, and a PhD in 1928 from the University of Illinois Department of Zoology. In the same year, he became assistant professor of zoology at Smith College, and soon after began his work at Clarke. Although he directed the school's heredity division for less than two years, he shaped its trajectory for decades. Hardly ever mentioned in accounts of Steggerda's life, his work at the school was an early manifestation of his meticulously detailed and tentative anthropology. Steggerda was an anthropologist in the broadest sense. Up to his early death in 1950, he undertook hundreds of longitudinal studies, recording a vast array of ethnographic, religious, anthropometric, hereditary, and psychological traits in populations as diverse as South American indigenous populations, Smith College and Clarke School students, Jamaicans, and his own extended family. He was noted for his extraordinarily meticulous, precise, and extensive records. More interested in describing and measuring traits than in analysing them, he left a vast archive that recently has drawn the attention of anthropologists, zoologists, and ethnologists.[11]

Steggerda's interest in the physical and mental variations between individuals, among races, and across populations brought him into contact with zoologist Charles Davenport, the director of the Eugenics Record Office. The two scientists met in 1926 and together undertook an extensive study of the native population of the West Indies. They published the results of their research in the 1928 *Race Crossing in Jamaica*, which detailed a huge array of physiological, psychological, and morphological traits in relation to the variability and supposed abilities of 'racial' hybrids.[12] Davenport and the ERO have become notorious as symbols of a racist, biased, deterministic, and coercive eugenics. Davenport's research, historian David Kevles writes, tended to 'incautious speculation', if not oversimplification and was based on a science 'that, even by standards of his own day, was usually dubious and often plain wrong'.[13] Other historians, however, have emphasized that his research was up to and contributed to the standards of his time – which certainly were, by our current standards, biased and racist. He turned the ERO into the central institution of American eugenics, promoted its methods and goals, and, not least, promoted research opportunities for an entire generation of scientists and fieldworkers, many of whom went on to influential positions elsewhere.[14]

In its set-up, the Clarke School heredity division shared many characteristics with the ERO, from collecting data through fieldwork and interviews to aggregating this data in pedigrees in the hope of finding simple Mendelian patterns. Their division of work between female staff members and male outside scientists also resembled that of the ERO. Between 1910 and 1924, the ERO trained 250 field workers – predominantly young, college-educated women – who travelled the country collecting traits of individuals and families in their homes, as well as in schools, hospitals, asylums, and other institutions. Like many middle-class women, these field workers were drawn to eugenics as a means for social reform through applied science. For some, their work for the ERO served as a springboard for careers in science, education, or social work.[15] Similar motives were at play for the two women involved with heredity research at the Clarke School, Ruth Pierce Guilder (1888–1945) and her assistant, the teacher and audiologist Louise A. Hopkins. With a BS from Simmons College and an MD from the University of Illinois, Guilder had worked as an editor for the American Medical Association before she came to the Clarke School in 1930. When, in the same year, Steggerda gave up his positions at Smith College and the Clarke School to become a full-time researcher at the ERO, Guilder took his position as head of the heredity division. This certainly was a step up from her editor job.[16]

Louise Hopkins' career, too, had a clear upward trajectory. After graduating from Buffalo Seminary and teaching high school maths, she had met Guilder while working at Sleighton Farms, an institution for 'delinquent' girls near Darlington, Pennsylvania. Why she decided to leave Sleighton Farms and come to work at the Clarke School is unclear, but in 1929 she graduated from Clarke's teacher-training programme and became Guilder's assistant in the heredity division. She worked there for the rest of her life, recording health and family data, and administering audiological tests to incoming and current students. When, in 1936, Guilder left the school due to health problems, Hopkins replaced her as head of the heredity research division. In 1939, she received a Master's degree in audiology from Massachusetts State College. Over the next decades, her position offered her the opportunity to interact with other researchers and to publish her work on hereditary deafness.[17]

The Clarke school's heredity division, however, was not simply a smaller version of the ERO. While the ERO engaged in extensive campaigns for negative and coercive eugenics, the school maintained Bell's reserve towards all forms of coercion. Venerating his achievements as a scientist and teacher, Clarke pursued a politics in which positive eugenics – encouraging good marriages – was integrated into the larger framework of oralist education. Nor did Steggerda simply imitate Davenport in setting up the division. More interested in observing and recording anthropological traits than in applied eugenics, he instilled in his co-workers a distinctly reserved stance when it came to drawing conclusions about hereditary patterns from their growing data collection.

The 'problem of inheritance of deafness', Ruth Guilder explained in 1932, 'must be approached from three angles: the genetic, the otological and the general medical'.[18] The school gathered such information in different ways. Just like the ERO field workers, Guilder and Hopkins visited students' families, inquiring about the incidence of deafness and other possibly connected traits. They also added new data to the pedigrees Bell had collected on Martha's Vineyard. Students' pedigrees were complemented with data from the children's medical records, kept and updated by Guilder and Hopkins in their double role as researchers and the school's health workers. Sometimes, children were admitted to the Evans Memorial Hospital in Boston 'for an exhaustive diagnostic study'.[19] If necessary, the school engaged outside experts, whose collaboration made the programme a multi-disciplinary and multi-institutional affair. Smith College zoologist Richard Post, for example, 'annually made anthropometric measurements of our pupils' to compare the growths of deaf and hearing children. Also involved were two Harvard scientists: Clyde E. Keeler, the university's first medical geneticist, who in 1921 was the first to link a nervous system defect to a single mutated gene, and Hallowell Davis, a pioneering neurophysiologist and leading authority on the ear and hearing.[20]

Audiology offered another, often more tangible and measurable angle to distinguish between different types of deafness. This was a relatively new approach. Audiometers – devices that measure the range of hearing by generating the respective range of sounds – had been developed soon after the invention of the telephone. Bell himself had constructed one of the first types, and Bell Telephone Laboratories later became an important manufacturer of audiometers. By the 1920s, the first electric models became available. It was in this decade, too, that the Clarke School purchased their first audiometer and, via their ties to Bell Telephone Laboratories, received custom-made models. Soon, extensive and repeated hearing tests became the school's standard. These audiological tests marked a shift away from the older practice of teachers' subjective evaluation of hearing loss towards the more objective and comparable audiograms.[21]

By the 1930s, researchers found uses for audiograms beyond determining educational placement. For his heredity research, William Tinkle, for example, compared audiograms of deaf parents with their hearing children to see whether one parent was able to perceive high, the other low tones. This would have indicated that deafness was caused by two different recessive genes, and explained why two deaf parents could have hearing and deaf children. No such distinctions could be found, however.[22] At the Clarke School, too, Hopkins and Guilder integrated pedigree information with individual audiograms, yet on a much larger scale. With this information they developed four different categories of hearing loss that 'served as a working base for both scientific and educational purposes'.[23] Just as an individual profile of hearing loss was the base for a successful oralist education, it was, Guilder wrote in 1933, 'in many ways the foundation for our research in the heredity of deafness'.[24] Thus both heredity and audiological research were to benefit the school in its quest to understand and prevent deafness and normalize its effects.

The 'devious ways in which deafness ... appears and disappears in the family tree': first results and competing analyses

In 1931, Steggerda, Guilder, and Hopkins presented their first *Report of the Research Department Concerning Heredity of Deafness*. Mainly a collection of hand-drawn pedigrees, divided into hereditary, non-hereditary, and mixed cases, it correlated deafness with data on birth date and place, death cause, and general health, noting characteristics such as 'Alcoholism', 'Tuberculosis', or 'Feeble-minded'. Rather cautiously, the report noted higher rates of hearing impairment in combination with tuberculosis, 'circulatory diseases', and 'suppurative ear condition'. Yet the limited analytic capacities of contemporary genetics allowed no judgement about whether these were environmental or hereditary cases. Rather than defining clearly identifiable patterns, the study mainly confirmed the belief that some forms of deafness indeed were hereditary. This finding, in turn, was underlined with general eugenic and oralist presumptions. Thus, pedigree four, an example of three generations of deafness 'illustrates the idea of "like marrying like"'. This, the authors warned, 'is a dangerous practice when the heredity of an abnormality is involved'.[25]

In the following years, research at Clarke followed a routine, as Guilder and Hopkins collected pedigree and medical information of incoming and current students. When Morris Steggerda left for a position at the ERO in 1930, Ruth Guilder took over his position. Her retirement in 1936 left Hopkins in charge of the division where, year for year, she meticulously collected pedigree, medical, and audiological information from the incoming students and their families. Yet what this growing data might mean remained unclear. To the Clarke School, results did little more than confirm the old concern about students passing on their condition. 'It is still too early', Guilder summarized in her last report, 'to undertake a detailed analysis or to determine the final significance of this material'.[26] Driven by an intense belief in the importance of learning about its students' genetic make-up, Clarke's heredity research was also marked by a distinct reluctance to draw any specific conclusions from its research data, other than a general disapproval of deaf intermarriage. This set the school apart from other research institutions in the eugenic area (and beyond), which were quick to claim clear patterns of inheritance for certain traits. Yet as time went on, it also made apparent the growing gap between the school's aspirations to be a leader in hereditary deafness research, and the changing state of the art outside the school's gates.

This did not mean that the Clarke School data did not contribute to a more sophisticated understanding of genetic deafness. The school's outside collaborators, more versed in genetic theory, and more embedded in academic research, were more decisive in their conclusion. These collaborations also make visible how different perceptions of eugenics, public health, and disability were crucial for how data was contextualized. The school's work with geneticist Madge T. Macklin during the 1940s provides another example. After Steggerda left, Clarke looked again for a scientist skilled in pedigree analysis, acknowledging that Hopkins had neither the training nor the skills for this task. The school hired Madge T. Macklin from the University of Western Ontario's medical faculty.[27] Macklin (1893–1962) was one of the few leading female scientists in the early history of genetics. In 1930, she was a cofounder of the Canadian Eugenics Society; from 1959 to 1960, she served as the first female president of the American Society for Human Genetics. Mostly known for her contributions to the heredity of cancers and other rare genetic conditions, Macklin's career belies the traditional periodization of a transition from racist, biased eugenics to medicalized human genetics.

For Macklin, eugenics was a form of preventive medicine; a means to improve public and individual health. Genetic knowledge, she believed, brought significant advantages to medical research and practice, improving differential diagnosis and, eventually, therapy. Awareness of a condition's hereditary character warranted prevention, both for the sake of public health and to limit individual suffering. To make these points, Macklin often used evocative, sometimes harsh eugenic language that subjugated the rights of supposedly genetically 'defective' individuals to a heroic vision of efficient disease eradication.[28] For Macklin, deafness exemplified the need for genetic knowledge as a means of prevention, and the Clarke School material offered an intriguing opportunity. The school gave her access to its vast collection of pedigrees and medical data, as well as the chance to educate an allegedly high-risk population group.

During the 1940s, when Macklin spent several vacations in Northampton, she and Hopkins systematized the Clarke material. This resulted in two publications: a two-part 1946 article in the *Laryngoscope*, co-authored by Hopkins and Macklin, and the more extensive 1949 *Clarke School Studies Concerning the Heredity of Deafness*.[29] These publications reflected their different approaches to hereditary deafness. For Macklin, shaped by her experience in medical and academic genetics, it was a clinical entity caused by specific, if as of yet unidentified genes. For Hopkins, grounded in the school's day-to-day life, it was a concerning, hard-to-grasp phenomenon that appeared, unexplained and disturbingly, in the student population. And where Macklin focused narrowly and from a distance on deafness as a matter of preventative medical genetics, Hopkins portrayed the school as an idealized, holistic institution in which education and research merged for the eugenic benefits of the research population and of science at large.

There was, Hopkins wrote, hardly any 'richer field for research' for hereditary deafness than the Clarke School, with its long tradition going back to Alexander Graham Bell. The school's 'old and very loyal alumni group, a considerable number of whom, unfortunately, have had deaf children to send back to the Clarke School' made multi-generational family studies possible. The school also had the 'absolute cooperation of the parents of our children, who are only too eager to do all in their power to help us in our efforts to learn more about the causes of deafness in childhood and the part played by inheritance in the production of deafness'.[30] The relationship between school, parents, and students, portrayed as harmonious, collaborative, and pursuing the same goal, characterized all school publications. How much this was true is hard to tell without parent and alumni narratives on heredity research. Recent investigations about physical abuse at Clarke during the 1950, 1960s, and 1970s, cast a strong doubt on such idealization, although this apparently did not involve the heredity division staff.[31] It is reasonable to assume that hearing parents – the majority – shared the school's interest in preventing hereditary deafness, in particular as research results might affect their own family planning. Deaf people, too, William Ennis has argued, had often internalized eugenic ideas about preventing deaf intermarriage and child-bearing, though often with some ambivalence.[32] This might have been particularly true for deaf parents who sent their children to Clarke, although in hindsight and with a lack of sources, we can only make assumptions about their private opinions.

Although Hopkins noted 'the devious ways in which deafness, even the so-called congenital deafness, appears and disappears in the family tree', she hesitated when it came to drawing conclusive, analytic results.[33] The 1949 *Clarke School Studies Concerning the Heredity of Deafness* presented pedigrees and complimentary material on 162-pages, with only a small part dedicated to summary and analysis. Hopkins believed that providing this 'data in full, without an analysis or commentary, will be more useful in the long run than committing ourselves at this time to the support of any particular hypothesis'. Instead, she called for the further cooperation between 'geneticists, otologists, auditory physicists and physicians' as the way to 'the final solution of the problem of heredity and its relation to deafness'.[34]

Macklin, on the other hand, teased out patterns of inheritance from data she acknowledged to be messy. Like Tinkle, she assumed that hereditary deafness was a recessive condition, with more than one gene responsible, although she could not distinguish these genes and their phenotypes. There was, she believed, a higher percentage of hereditary deafness than often assumed. When, for example, a deaf child was born in a family with no recorded history of hearing loss, parents and physicians often attributed deafness to infectious diseases, even if more deaf siblings were born. Recessive inheritance could explain these occurrences, and according to Macklin was responsible for up to two thirds of such sporadic cases. Heredity, then, was an invisible risk, looming even over individuals previously considered unaffected. Keeping with the theme of an invisible genetic state, she suggested 'that a child may be genotypically deaf, but phenotypically hearing'. Similar to a diabetic who did not yet show signs of disease, a 'deaf person might be genetically deaf but still have enough hearing to pass for a hearing person'. This was consistent with the Clarke School often finding some level of hearing loss in hearing family members of deaf students. For Macklin, these were examples for the benefits of genetic knowledge – and the dangers of remaining ignorant. Only with such knowledge one could look beyond a temporary phenotypical state and recognize an individual's true, genetic nature – their medical fate.[35]

The need for prevention and the urgency to promote genetic awareness were common denominators between Hopkins and Macklin. Yet where Macklin was rooted in the world of academic science, of proving or disproving certain theories, Hopkins saw the students she worked with over the years, their families, and their future children, who they perhaps would send back to the school. And where Macklin sought genes and disease patterns, for Hopkins, the pedigrees, with their multiple cases of congenital deafness, confirmed older fears about the dangers of deaf intermarriage. In turn, these different preconceptions would also shape heredity counselling.

Counselling, education, and prevention: applied heredity research

Like with almost all genetic conditions, knowledge in the 1940s was insufficient to definitely identify a person as genetically deaf, or to predict whether a couple would pass on their deafness. At 'the present time', Hopkins admitted, 'we do not have enough knowledge to make accurate predictions possible'.[36] Yet at the Clarke School, hereditary deafness was never only an abstract trait tracked for academic pursuit, but something that staff and teachers observed in their daily work with their students. Teachers, Hopkins reported, were faced with difficult questions: 'What advice shall be given a former pupil who is contemplating marriage with a former deaf classmate? What can we say to the hearing brothers and sisters when they ask whether they may have deaf children if they marry?' Parents, too, felt responsible to explain to their children that their condition might be passed on.[37]

Despite, or perhaps just because of, the vague nature of hereditary deafness, the school felt responsible for providing students and their families with an awareness of their (assumed) genetic status. For each student, the division kept a comprehensive folder. It consisted of a family pedigree, consecutive otological and audiometric reports, and the student's medical history, ideally from birth, but certainly since his or her entry into the school.[38] This material was used in a multitude of ways that combined research, counselling, and oralist education. As Guilder put it in 1932, the division hoped that eventually 'we may be of greater assistance to the teachers through our studies of the individual child'.[39] In particular the school's use of audiological profiles demonstrates how closely intertwined were the short-term goals of special education and the long-term goals of heredity research. An audiogram was not only indicative of a student's educational needs and potential. Together with their medical file and pedigree, it also could give hints for diagnosis of a specific type of deafness. Together with other family members' audiograms, it placed the student into an intergenerational network, and provided the staff with information for reducing the impact of deafness on the educational, medical, and genetic level.

For this purpose, students of the graduating class received a 'demonstration and interpretation of family charts'. This group, prepared for further education, marriage, or professional life by years of rigorous oral education, now received additional, hereditary advice. 'Upon request', Guilder reported, 'those who wished it were given an opportunity for individual conferences'.[40] Whether or not these were mandatory was not noted, though presumably participation was at least recommended, if not expected. Through such activities, heredity research, education, and practical eugenics merged.[41] How students reacted to this advice, and whether they followed it, was not noted. As with the principles of oralist education in general, Clarke expected compliancy, yet did not publicly note non-compliant behaviour – not least because doing so would have revealed the limits of their influence on students' life choices after graduation. However, there is no indication that heredity education had a noticeable impact on the rates of deaf intermarriage. If there had ever been any doubt that Clarke School alumni married each other or found deaf spouses elsewhere, the school's very own heredity research made clear that this was and remained common.

In the 1940s, the school was among a growing number of institutions that offered heredity counselling. Combining genetic advice, education, and research, the school shared some important qualities with these heredity clinics. Usually linked to medical schools or university hospitals, they were founded by leading geneticists. They were a link between the more public health-oriented, state-guided eugenics of the 1920s and 1930s and the professionalizing, university-based medical genetics that emerged from the 1940s on. By attaching heredity clinics to medical schools, their founders hoped to integrate genetics more closely with medical practice and education, and to promote good eugenic behaviour. They pursued the medical-eugenic goal of preventing disease, defects, and suffering at the individual and the population level. For the most part, heredity clinics distanced themselves from coercive eugenic measures such as sterilization legislation or marriage restrictions, instead pursuing a politics of persuasive education and counselling – at least for the part of the population they considered capable of making such reasonable decisions. In this, they shared with the Clarke School the belief that once adequately educated on genetic risk, the desire for a 'normal' family and a 'normal' child would guide reproductive decisions.[42] They also shared the conviction that professionals in education or social work, too, needed to have a basic awareness of genetic mechanisms, so they could recognize hereditary patterns. For this purpose, the Clarke School also provided lectures on hereditary deafness to teachers in training.

While the school had much common with heredity clinics, much separated them. Heredity clinics operated in a context of academic science, clinical medicine, and outpatient counselling. Their educational mission was limited to spreading awareness of genetic conditions and imbuing a sense of genetic responsibility in clients who were seen a few times at best. Applied heredity research at the Clarke School, on the other hand, took place at a residential school where the research staff was personally familiar with their research objects. They observed students over many years, got to know their families, and followed their post-graduation careers.

In her role as the school's audiologist, health worker, and heredity researcher, Louise Hopkins was dedicated as much to oralist education as to the more abstract eugenic effects of their research. This familiarity with students and dedication to an oralist framework closely shaped counselling and the perception of genetic risk. Compared to the medical-eugenic mission of the heredity clinics, the school pursued a much wider, more holistic goal: the formation of a well-rounded deaf citizen who succeeded socially and professionally in hearing society. All of the school's research was to contribute to this goal. Just as the psychology division would improve educational theory and practice, and just as phonetic research would improve the efficiency of oralist schooling, so would heredity research enable 'normal' family life for future generations. With heredity research, this remained much more a vision than a reality, yet this did not diminish the staff's sense of purpose and urgency.

Eugenicists' focus on biological limits and educators' emphasis of human malleability have often been considered incompatible. Historian Diane Paul concluded that hereditary determinism contradicted the American belief in education and experience: 'Eugenicists', she wrote, 'had to counter the powerful American faith in education and in the efficacy of moral effort'.[43] The Clarke School, however, reconciled both strands. Unlike educators for the 'feeble-minded', the school never propagated an image of the deaf as unsuited for marriage or incapable of raising children. Rather, married family life was an attribute of the normal citizenship the school envisioned for their students. In this sense, the school's reproductive policy resembled the pro-natalist strand of eugenics that contributed to the idealization of family and marriage in the 1940s and 1950s.[44] From the standpoint of an oralist school, a good marriage was that of a deaf to a hearing person, signalling successful integration into society.

It was thus not (hereditary) hearing status that implied a deaf person's worth, but their ability to overcome their disability through the laborious effort of learning oral communication and of thus passing as 'normal'. Hard work, the school never tired of repeating, was rewarded with acceptance by and success in hearing society. Assessing a child – and by extension their family – for hereditary deafness did not necessarily change this set of values. Within the larger scheme of eliminating (the effects of) deafness, it was yet another new and promising tool to prevent or even eliminate deafness in future generations. Heredity advice provided students with the knowledge to make good, rational decisions in yet another realm, enabling them to continue their trajectory as successfully integrated citizens. In this manner, the medicalization and technologization of deafness went hand in hand with redefining who a deaf person could and should become.

As oralism promised normalization – increasingly aided by assistive technology – it left little room for identities beyond this strongly medicalized and pathologizing frame. Residential schools established an all-encompassing environment that patrolled social, moral, linguistic, and reproductive behaviour. The school's ideal of the oralized deaf citizen severely restricted the meaning of 'good' behaviour, defining as deviant or 'defective' the deaf person who did not learn to speak and lip-read sufficiently, and who could not (or did not want to) pass as hearing. This was always as much an ideal as a reality. Not least the school's own psychological research under Fritz and Grace Moore Heider had shown that after graduation, many Clarke School students joined the signing deaf community, and had little contact with the hearing world. Yet when it came to marriage and founding a family, such behaviour was seen as more than a matter of individual failure. Marrying another deaf person had taken on strong undertones of eugenic irresponsibility, of not only bringing harm to oneself, but potentially to one's children and to society at large.

Big science at a small school: the promises of medical genetics

In 1959, after three decades of administering hearing tests and collecting pedigrees, of corresponding with fellow genetic deafness researchers all over the world and publishing in various scientific journals, Louise Hopkins retired.[45] She urged the school to publish the data she had accumulated: 'No other school for the deaf or research center has as much material on heredity of deafness. It should not remain locked away in our files'.[46] School officials agreed.

Hopkins' successor as head of the heredity division was the teacher Ruth B. Hudgins (1907–2009). She was the wife of Clarence W. Hudgins, who led the division of experimental phonetics, and from 1960 directed the research department as a whole. Ruth Hudgins' background – early aspirations to be a classical pianist, an undergraduate degree from Oberlin College, and a MEd from Smith College – suggested little to recommend her for heredity research.[47] The same, of course, had been true for Louise Hopkins, when she became Guilder's assistant in 1929. Yet in the era of eugenic fieldworkers, the school's practice of recruiting teachers as research staff had been nothing unusual, and in fact was an established practice. Thirty years later, in a drastically changed and professionalized landscape of genetic research, it marked Clarke's falling out of time. Consequently, Hudgins tasks and involvement remained more limited than Hopkins'. She took over Hopkins' routine of collecting pedigrees and medical information, as well as her position as school nurse who chronicled the students' health, and administered vaccinations, vision tests, or fluoride tablets.[48] Yet unlike Hopkins, she did not carve out a role for herself in the larger world of genetic deafness research, however small.

The school followed Hopkins' plea to publish her accumulated material. Once more, they looked for a scientist to guide analysis, and eventually found him in the young biochemical geneticist Kenneth Brown (1929–2015). Brown had received a BA from the University of Michigan Department of Zoology in

1949 and an MD from its medical school in 1960. Other than a brief hospital internship, he was never really a practising physician; he was more interested in biochemical and population genetics than in its clinical application. In 1961, when Clarke tried to engage him, he was just about to take a position as clinical associate at the Human Genetics Section of the NIH Institute of Dental Research (NIDR). Under its head Carl Witkop (1920–1993), a pioneer of oral and dental genetics, the NIDR investigated a broad range of genetic phenomena.[49]

Brown's interest in deafness had only been peripheral so far. But like with Steggerda and Macklin, the Clarke School data offered an intriguing research opportunity. He shared with Steggerda an interest in population research, although human population sciences had changed quite a bit since Steggerda's time. Steggerda, the broadly educated anthropologist, had collected an almost infinite variety of physical, social, and cultural traits, but was more interested in the collection than the analysis. Brown, on the other hand, was a biomedical scientist, who analysed and correlated pedigrees, blood, and tissue samples with the aid of laboratory techniques and computerized statistics in order to find underlying biochemical mechanisms.

More generally, the landscape of American science and science funding had been changing rapidly. The 'big science' that emerged in the aftermath of World War II grew not least because of expanding federal funding, and, in the US, was institutionalized with the foundation of the NIH. Biomedical science now required expansive laboratory space and expensive equipment, highly specialized scientists, and a supporting network of laboratory staff and administrators.[50]

The changed landscape of biomedical research impacted the terms of collaboration between the Clarke School and outside researchers. With Steggerda and Macklin, the school had determined the extent of research and the manner of publication. Brown, on the other hand, took charge from the beginning, and brought in the NIH's impressive resources and staff. Arriving at the NIH in 1961, he discovered that a group of scientists there was already working on deafness. George Cassady, a senior paediatrics resident at Harvard Medical School, and geneticist Maimon Cohen, a junior assistant health service officer at the NIH, had initiated a biochemical study of genetic deafness and renal dysfunction (Alport syndrome). Their work at the intersection between the laboratory and the clinic was typical for the course of genetics in the 1960s, requiring ever greater resources and specialization. By October 1961, Brown had joined Cassady's and Cohen's project, and suggested combining research at Clarke with NIH resources.[51]

Obligated to school traditions, Hudgins had originally planned to simply publish the accumulated pedigrees in a format like the 1949 monograph: descriptive rather than analytical. Eventually, however, he agreed to Brown's much more expansive plan. In 1962, the cooperation between the Clarke School, the NIDR, and the National Institute of Neurological Diseases and Blindness was formalized. With a budget of $54,440 over the course of four and a half years, the project's goal was to differentiate subtypes of genetic deafness, and to establish correlations with other conditions. The project started in late 1962 and lasted until 1966. The research team saw one unexpected addition: Louise Hopkins returned from retirement, providing her intimate knowledge of the material. During the project, the researchers assessed existing pedigrees, sent out 3,500 questionnaires to former students, and visited families to conduct interviews and physical examinations, investigating, among other things, eye, heart, and thyroid conditions associated with hearing loss.[52]

New and existing material together amounted to an ever-growing bulk of data that was beyond the analytic capacities of any single scientist. New insights to the genetic mechanisms of deafness also complicated analysis. By the 1950s, researchers had realized that there needed to be more than only a few genes to account for the complex and diverse patterns of inheritance found with deafness. They believed that there was a much larger number of recessive, dominant, or sex-linked forms, some of which were non-syndromic, others inherited together with other traits. Consequently, finding a seemingly clear pattern of inheritance in one family's pedigree did not necessarily mean that it applied to another. Even in the same family, hearing loss could be caused by different genes, or could be genetic in some members and environmental in others.[53]

In the early 1960s, there was a new and promising approach for tackling these increasingly complex constellations: computerized data analysis. In genetics, computerized statistics made possible significant progress in following the segregation and linkage of traits in large populations, and thus to see whether (and how many) distinct genes were responsible. In deafness research in particular, advanced computing would make a real impact. It enabled scientists to tackle enormous sets of population data such as the Clarke School material, in order to identify patterns of inheritance and their frequency in a population, and to speculate about underlying genes. Reversely, genetic counselling could then draw from such population statistics for more refined prognoses with an individual or a couple, or to identify unaffected carriers in a family.[54]

The NIH was an important forerunner in biomedical computing, making it possible for Brown to use this new technology for the Clarke School data. Planning to transfer their material to punch cards – the preferred data storage medium in early computing – he brought in his colleague Chin Sik Chung, an expert in the computerized analysis of genetic data. Born in Korea in 1924, Chung had received a PhD in genetics from the University of Wisconsin, Madison in 1957 before moving on to the NIH in 1961.[55] Chung had belonged to the team that had first used a computer program for a sophisticated segregation analysis of genetic deafness. In 1959, he and population geneticist Newton E. Morton had published a statistical study of Northern Ireland – a region small enough that the entire deaf population had been ascertained. They concluded that autosomal recessive inheritance was responsible for about 68 per cent of all genetic cases, with up to thirty-six genes involved. Autosomal dominant inheritance, with at least two gene defects, made up 22 per cent. The remaining 9 per cent, the authors ascribed to 'sporadic cases, due to unrecognized infection or more complex genetic mechanisms'.[56] These sophisticated results, obtained with the help of computerized segregation analysis, made the Northern Ireland study a trendsetter for the direction of genetic deafness research in the 1960s and 1970s.

Applying computerized statistics to the Clarke School material, Brown and Chung came to somewhat different conclusions. The Northern Ireland study assumed that the estimated thirty-six recessive genes were about equally frequent, and thus rare. If this was the case, it was unlikely that two deaf parents had the same gene. Consequently, the number of deaf children resulting from such marriages should be very low. This was not the case with the Clarke School data, however, where there were eighty-seven sibships from marriages, in which at least one parent was a former student. This was only possible if there was a lower and unevenly distributed number of recessive genes. Brown and Chung gave an estimate of five common genes and 'many more rare genes causing deafness'.[57] Reversely, assuming that genes for deafness were both numerous and, mostly, rare, explained why sometimes, two (presumably) genetically deaf parents from families with many deaf members had mostly or only hearing children. These insights would have important consequences for genetic counselling.

What about deaf intermarriage? New insights and new advice

When it ended in 1966, the collaboration between the Clarke School and the NIH had brought together two very different partners. It had made visible the school's change in status from a leading centre of genetic deafness research in the 1930s and 1940s to a location for fieldwork. It also made visible both a renewed belief in the scientific manageability of deafness, and a growing disconnect in the way geneticists and educators conceptualized genetic deafness, and in what they considered good advice about marriage and reproduction.

Advances in understanding genetic deafness brought together more closely diagnosis, prevention, and hope for therapy. Research of syndromic deafness in particular shows these increasingly close ties between medicine, genetics, and genetic counselling. Deafness is sometimes inherited together with a number of other metabolic conditions (e.g. Pendred syndrome), with craniofacial or skeletal malformations (e.g. Wildervanck syndrome) or pigmentation changes (Waardenburg syndrome). A handful of these, for example hereditary deaf-blindness (Usher syndrome), were already known, to some degree, in the late nineteenth and early twentieth century. But it was only in the 1950s that research of syndromic deafness proliferated. Looking at a pedigree and following distinct, often visible traits associated with deafness, such as the differently coloured eyes and white forelock characteristic for Waardenburg syndrome, had distinct advantages. In this manner, patterns of inheritance could be established even without understanding the underlying biochemical or chromosomal mechanisms. Research of syndromic forms also brought together more closely genetics with medical practice, as with the NIH project on renal disease and deafness (Alport syndrome), or Brown and Chung's survey of deafness and thyroid and heart disease at the Clarke School.[58]

The realization that a significant number of genetically deaf individuals might be affected by undiagnosed kidney, heart, or thyroid conditions brought a new kind of urgency to debates about detection and prevention. It strengthened the notion that genetic deafness was a condition calling for close medical supervision. This was a relatively new idea. Before the 1950s, surveying an individual or population for hereditary deafness had been mostly a matter of eugenic prevention in the coming generation. For mid-century geneticists, however, it also became a medical concern for the current generation. Alport syndrome, for example, demonstrated the urgency for early diagnosis so the renal dysfunction could be treated. Although it 'might represent a significant disease among the deaf', Brown explained in 1964, it had been neglected.[59] Similarly, English otologist Ladislav Fisch urged in 1963 that the old, laconic assessment 'cause of deafness unknown' was no longer acceptable. He elaborated: '*careful clinical examination will often discover minimal expression of a genetic condition* and so identify the true nature of the hearing loss'.[60] By contrasting present neglect with the possibilities of biomedical research, Brown, Fisch, and others created a sense of urgency, in which applied genetics became a matter of responsibility towards a population threatened by genetic disease.

To geneticists, this increasingly close connection between diagnosis, (potential) therapy, and prevention demonstrated the need for genetic record-keeping, education, and counselling. The Clarke School, Brown explained at an NIH conference in 1964, 'illustrates the advantage of a register system with a well-documented population'. He 'encouraged conference participants to start to collect pedigrees', ensuring them that 'it does not require a high degree of sophistication'. Their analysis of the Clarke School data, he added with some hyperbole, 'presented the first opportunity to give soundly based scientific information to deaf people who are contemplating marriage with other deaf people'. This, the conference report added, 'of course, is a common situation'.[61]

Research of syndromic deafness also impacted reproductive counselling. In a time before genetic testing, syndromic traits offered a means to diagnose specific subforms in individuals, and thus to predict the reproductive outcome between two persons. No longer generally disapproving of deaf intermarriage, geneticists now were optimistic that they could provide more individualized reproductive counselling. Dutch geneticist-physician L. S. Wildervanck for example explained at the 1963 annual Convention of American Instructors of the Deaf that the likelihood of a deaf couple carrying the same gene for hearing loss was low. 'There is no reason', he commented, 'to discourage a marriage between individuals respectively suffering from the common recessively inherited deafness and deafness belonging to a hereditary syndrome'.[62]

Wildervanck's optimism about prognosis and his narrow focus on reproductive outcomes were typical for the pro-natalist stance of contemporary American genetics, which portrayed itself as a science enabling rather than restricting marriage and 'normal' family life. Not everybody, however, was ready to give up the old cautionary stance on deaf intermarriage: summarizing the contributions to a 1967 conference on *Deafness in Childhood*, renowned otolaryngologist George E. Shambaugh noted that 'Dr. Brown's chapter [on genetic deafness] is most interesting'. He felt 'encouraged by the fact that two deaf parents could expect to have 60 percent normal hearing children'. Nevertheless, he maintained, 'I still would not encourage two deaf people to marry if they are congenitally deaf'.[63] The old oralist suspicion of deaf intermarriage, tangled with social belief and moral judgement, was hard to dismiss.

Wildervanck's and Shambaugh's opinions signalled the slow unravelling of the coalition between geneticists and oralist educators. It had formed in the aftermath of A. G. Bell's *Memoir*, and at the Clarke School had been strengthened in the 1930s and 1940s. By the 1950s, however, ever more specialized perceptions of deafness in different professions resulted in diverging notions of risk, pathology, or failure. While geneticists focused narrowly on 'normal' reproductive outcomes, to oralist educators the reproduction of normalcy and the 'normal' family encompassed something much bigger: a holistic ideal of training deaf children to pass as hearing in every aspect of their lives. In this context, deaf intermarriage continued to signify potential failure. In some sense, then, by mid-century genetic counselling for deafness became less restrictive, no longer automatically disapproving of deaf intermarriage – if provided in a medical-genetic context, rather than in an oralist school. Nevertheless, even though they came to disagree about what to advise, both geneticists and educators still agreed that deafness was a grave disability to be cured, prevented, or overcome.

Conclusion

The founding and funding of Clarke's research department was a prime example for a progressive era science project financed by private philanthropic charity. More or less wealthy private donors had given their money in exchange for taking part in a secularized salvation of the 'deserving disabled' through science. During the first two decades of research, the school was able to attract important figures from various scientific fields – Kurt Koffka or Fritz Heider for psychology, Morris Steggerda or Madge Macklin for heredity research – who considered the school an interesting research partner. With these resources and its contacts, the school became the primary site of American genetic deafness research during the 1930s and 1940s, drawing attention from researchers all over the world. Yet while work at Clarke's heredity division went on in the same manner decade after decade, biomedical research beyond the school walls changed rapidly and irrevocably. By the middle of the twentieth century, a small school with moderate resources and without trained scientists could no longer manage to be involved in basic research in several fields. School officials recognized this, too, and in the 1960s gradually moved away from basic research and towards investing into audiology and speech therapy services. This strategy worked well for maintaining Clarke's 'role as a leader among oral schools', as their centenary report claimed.[64] For the school, this was not so much a change in status as a change in focus. It continued to promote an image of Clarke as a place where the newest scientific research was applied to individualized education to 'overcome' deafness. This was as much rhetoric as reality, as the work of the heredity or psychology division made clear. Yet in the world of both deaf education and science funding, it remained a highly appealing rhetoric.

The school's heredity research could not keep up to date with the move towards large-scale, specialized laboratory and clinical research within genetics. When, in the 1960s, Kenneth Brown came to the school, he treated Clarke as a site for fieldwork rather than an independent research centre. This increasing divide between educators and biomedical scientists was not only one of staff, resources, and lab equipment, but also of approaches to genetic deafness and counselling. Oralist educators and geneticists had long agreed that deaf people should not marry each other. Now, though, geneticists began to take a less restrictive stance. They did so with a growing confidence in their ability to predict reproductive outcomes, and with a more permissive attitude towards the reproductive agency of their clients. Eager to demonstrate that their science was a democratic one that enabled rather than restricted family life, they actually encouraged deaf intermarriage, if the two people involved were unlikely to have the same type of deafness, and thus would not pass on their deafness. With this more permissive stance, they increasingly found themselves out of sync with oralist educators, who continued to expect assimilation to hearing norms in professional, private, marital, and reproductive life. In the setting of an oralist school, deaf intermarriage was an educational and social, if not a moral problem, a matter of non-compliance.

Among historians and geneticists, there has been an ongoing debate on whether and to what extent eugenic thought and motives persisted into the 1950s and 1960s. The Clarke School shows that the need to distance oneself from the 'old', bad and coercive eugenics depended on what heredity research and its practical eugenic applications had meant in first place. For the school, it had always been clear that their students did not belong to the same class of 'defectives' targeted by sterilization legislation or other coercive forms of eugenic. In a way, the school had always relied on non-coercive, persuasive forms of hereditary advice, which in the 1940s and 1950s became the new paradigm. Like the genetic counselling of the 1950s, it was based on the assumption that the informed individual would come to the 'right' reproductive decision once educated on their genetic make-up. However, non-directive counselling demanded (at least in theory) that professionals should not influence client decisions. The school, on the other hand, continued to operate with a persuasive paternalism that assumed medical and cultural agency over students. Just as teachers steered them away from the conspicuous use of sign language and other expressions of deaf difference, they aimed to instil a sense of responsibility for preventing deafness in future generations.

The effects of this counselling on individual attitudes remain unclear. School publications and communications habitually ignored behaviour they considered deviant, such as signing or joining the deaf community. More generally, it has been difficult to measure the effect of eugenic thought on the marriages and reproduction of white, working or middle-class deaf people, that is, those deaf people who were not threatened by coercive eugenic measures because of their race, gender, poverty, or disabilities. Historians of genetics have pointed to the long-lasting influences of eugenic ideals on marriage and child-bearing, not least because they resonated with larger ideas about ability and citizenship. Historians of deafness have argued that eugenic rhetoric from teachers and deaf leaders affected the community's attitudes to deaf intermarriage and preferences for deaf or hearing children.[65] However, at least at the Clarke School, the rates of deaf intermarriage among former students seemed to remain constant over the decades, and, ironically, continued to provide useful data for heredity research. As Kenneth Brown stated in 1970, 'a large proportion of Clarke School alumni got married often with their school alumni'.[66] In their 1960s study, which also looked at whether students had hearing or deaf parents, in almost 28 per cent of 832 marriages both parents were deaf. Unlike for the school, for Brown, these intermarriages were no reason for concern, but provided important information for analysing the number of different genes involved.

Nevertheless, even if the school's counselling apparently failed its goal, heredity research had an unacknowledged irony that endangered the very normalcy it claimed for its students. The school's foundational mission was to prove the inherent normalcy of deaf people, their potential to achieve an all-around 'normal' life. This was not only an educational achievement, but increasingly also one of science and medicine, an area in which the school considered itself a pioneer. Yet by engaging in research, the school anxiously tried to determine what, in first place, made their students different. With heredity research, this meant revealing an underlying trait that would limit their normalcy in marriage and reproduction. Normalization, then, relied heavily on medicalization; and heredity research very much operated within this tension of medicalization and normalization, of detecting and (potentially) correcting defects.

For professionals, advocating ever-earlier interventions to correct – or even prevent – deviance from the norm was a way to overcome this tension between defining and normalizing pathology. In the 1960s, audiologists, educators, and geneticists pushed for ever-earlier, even pre-natal identification of hearing loss by various (not necessarily reliable) means, such as maternal ultrasound or new-born screening.[67] Mid-century genetics was part of this mantra of early diagnosis and prevention. Genetic diagnosis was no longer only a matter of preventing deafness in the next generation. With research of syndromic deafness came the realization that a great number of traits and conditions – some grave, some non-pathological – were inherited along with hearing loss. This knowledge strengthened the push for early diagnosis, and added a new dimension to the medicalization of deafness. No longer was the deaf child only to be treated for hearing loss, now he or she also needed to be monitored for renal or cardiac disease, vision loss, or metabolic conditions.

What continued to unite geneticists and educators, then, was the firm and paternalistic belief in their ability to fix deafness and disability through scientific progress. Genetic deafness research remained a field in which hearing professionals defined problems and applied scientific solutions to an abstracted population. In a period in which the demarcation between hearing professionals and deaf people was still almost absolute, the latter featured in professional publications or conferences mainly as idealizations of oralist success or as depersonalized medical cases. That there was a world of signing deaf adults was something that oralist educators knew, but decided to silently ignore, and that consequently did not enter professional consciousness. Physicians or geneticists, whose contact with deaf people was sporadic and limited to clinical encounters, often were actually unaware of deaf culture and community. By the late 1950s, however, this one-sided and paternalistic perspective came to be challenged. As researchers began working with deaf, signing adults, long-held beliefs about the nature and meaning of deafness began to shift.

Notes

1 For continuities and reorientation among American eugenicists and geneticists see e.g. A. M. Stern, *Eugenic Nation: Faults and Frontiers of Better Breeding in Modern America* (Berkeley, CA: University of California Press, 2005), pp. 115–79; M. Ladd-Taylor, 'Eugenics, sterilisation and modern marriage in the USA: the strange career of Paul Popenoe', *Gender and History*, 13:2 (2001), 298–327; Kline, *Better Race*, pp. 124–56; Comfort, *Human Perfection*, pp. 67–129.
2 See e.g. N. Roll-Hansen, 'The progress of eugenics: growth of knowledge and change in ideology', *History of Science*, 26 (1988), 295–331.
3 Best, *The Deaf*, pp. 17, 41–2; Johnson, *Standardization*, p. 204.
4 Best, *The Deaf*, p. 41.
5 E. A. Fay, *Marriages of the Deaf in America: An Inquiry Concerning the Results of Marriages of the Deaf in America* (Washington, DC: Gibson bros., printers and bookbinders, 1898), p. 132. For Fay's beliefs about marital happiness see p. 135.
6 *Ibid.*, pp. 129–33.
7 For Mendelism as a guiding paradigm of genetics see G. E. Allen, 'The Eugenics Record Office at Cold Spring Harbor, 1910–1940: an essay in institutional history', *Osiris 2nd series*, 2 (1986), 225–64, here 239–40; Comfort, *Human Perfection*, pp. 1–28.
8 R. Linneaus, 'Heredity and intermarriage', *Volta Review*, 14 (1912), 184–6, here 184.
9 W. J. Tinkle, 'Deafness as a eugenical problem' (doctoral dissertation, Ohio State University, 1932). Tinkle, who rejected evolution, later wrote a creationist eugen-

ics textbook and in the 1960s played a significant role in the creationist movement. See R. L. Numbers, *The Creationists* (New York: A. A. Knopf, 1992), pp. 222–4.
10 W. J. Tinkle, 'Deafness as a eugenic problem', *Journal of Heredity*, 24 (1933), 13–18, here 14, 18.
11 A book-length biography of Steggerda remains to be written. For an overview see P. S. Sledzik, 'The Morris Steggerda Human Biology Collection', *National Museum of Health and Medicine, Armed Forces Institute of Pathology, Washington, DC, USA, Ethnographical Series*, 20 (2001), 281–6.
12 C. B. Davenport and M. Steggerda, *Race Crossing in Jamaica* (Washington, DC: Carnegie Institution of Washington, 1929).
13 D. J. Kevles, *In the Name of Eugenics: Genetics and the Uses of Human Heredity: With a New Preface by the Author* (Cambridge, MA: Harvard University Press, 1997), p. 48.
14 See Allen, 'The Eugenics Record Office', 226–8, 240.
15 See Paul, *Controlling Human Heredity*, pp. 51–7; A. S. Bix, 'Experiences and voices of eugenics field-workers: "women's work" in biology', *Social Studies of Science*, 27:4 (1997), 625–68.
16 Special Collections and University Archives, Umass Amherst Libraries, Clarke School for the Deaf (MS 742), 'Biographical file Ruth Guilder'.
17 Special Collections and University Archives, Umass Amherst Libraries, Clarke School for the Deaf (MS 742), 'Biographical file, Hopkins, Louise Alice'. For her thesis see L A. Hopkins, 'The influence of the type of audiogram upon the child's ability to interpret speech sounds' (MS thesis, Massachusetts State College Amherst, 1939).
18 R. Guilder, 'Report of the research department', *Clarke School Annual Report*, 65 (1932), 25–9, here 25.
19 Numbers, *My Words Fell on Deaf Ears*, p. 101.
20 *Ibid.*, p. 104.
21 *Ibid.*, pp. 81, 101. For the history of audiometers see S. D. Stephens, 'Audiometers from Hughes to modern times', *British Journal of Audiology, Supplement*, 2 (1979), 17–23.
22 Tinkle, 'Deafness as a eugenic problem', 15–16.
23 Numbers, *My Words Fell on Deaf Ears*, p. 102.
24 R. Guilder, 'Report of the research department', *Clarke School Annual Report*, 66 (1933), 35–40, here 36.
25 M. Steggerda, R. Guilder, and L. A. Hopkins, *Report of the Research Department Concerning Heredity of Deafness* (Northampton, MA: Clarke School for the Deaf, 1931), p. 90.
26 R. Guilder, 'Report of the research department', *Clarke School Annual Report*, 70 (1937), 27–9, here 27.
27 See F. H. Reiter, 'Report of the principal', *Clarke School Annual Report*, 72 (1939), 17–22.
28 For Macklin's position in contemporary eugenics and genetics see N. C. Comfort,

"'Polyhybrid heterogeneous bastards": promoting medical genetics in America in the 1930s and 1940s', *Journal of the History of Medicine and Allied Sciences*, 61 (2006), 415–55, here 415, 432–7.

29 See L. A. Hopkins, 'Studies on the inheritance of deafness in the pupils of the Clarke School for the Deaf: the collection of family histories, pedigrees and audiometer readings', *The Laryngoscope*, 56:10 (1946), 570–82; M. T. Macklin, 'Studies on the inheritance of deafness in the pupils of the Clarke School for the Deaf: genetic analysis of data and pedigrees', *The Laryngoscope*, 56:10 (1946), 583–601. The 1949 monograph only acknowledges Macklin and instead posthumously names Ruth Guilder as one of the authors. See L. A. Hopkins and R. P. Guilder, *Clarke School Studies Concerning the Heredity of Deafness: Pedigree Data 1930-1940* (Northampton, MA: Clarke School for the Deaf, 1949).

30 Hopkins, 'Studies', 571–2.

31 See Christensen, '"In a glass box"'.

32 See Ennis, 'Hereditarian ideas'.

33 Hopkins, 'Studies', 571.

34 Hopkins and Guilder, *Clarke School Studies*, pp. iii–iv.

35 Macklin, 'Studies', 586–7, 596–7. For Macklin's theories of complex inheritance see Comfort, '"Polyhybrid heterogeneous bastards"', 438.

36 Hopkins and Guilder, *Clarke School Studies*, p. iv.

37 Hopkins, 'Studies', 570.

38 *Ibid.*, 575.

39 Guilder, 'Report of the research department' (1932), 28.

40 Guilder, 'Report of the research department' (1937), 28, 29.

41 L. A. Hopkins, 'Report of the research department', *Clarke School Annual Report*, 71 (1940), 37–43, here 41.

42 For the history of the heredity clinics see Comfort, *Human Perfection*, pp. 97–127; Stern, *Telling Genes*, pp. 7–27; Ladd-Taylor, '"A kind of genetic social work"'; R. Resta, 'The historical perspective: Sheldon Reed and 50 years of genetic counseling', *Journal of Genetic Counseling*, 6:4 (1996), 375–7.

43 Paul, *Controlling Human Heredity*, p. 11.

44 See Kline, *Better Race*, pp. 124–56.

45 See L. A. Hopkins and L. G. Kinzer, 'Comparison of a group of rubella-deafened children with a group of hereditarily deaf children and their sibs', *American Journal of Diseases of Children*, 78:2 (1949), 182–200; L. A. Hopkins and R. Post, 'Deafmutism in two pairs of identical twins', *Journal of Heredity*, 47:2 (1956), 88–90; L. A. Hopkins, 'Heredity and deafness', *Eugenics Quarterly*, 1:3 (1954), 193–9.

46 L. A. Hopkins, 'Report of the research department', *Clarke School Annual Report*, 92 (1959), 64–7, here 67.

47 G. T. Pratt, 'Report of the principal', *Clarke School Annual Report*, 93 (1960), 21–39. For Ruth Hudgins career see her obituary, Anon., 'Ruth Hudgins, 101, Teacher, Music Lover', *Daily Hampshire Gazette* (29 April 2009).

48 See R. Hudgins, 'Division concerning the heredity of deafness', *Clarke School Annual Report*, 93 (1960), 33–5.
49 Anon., 'Kenneth Stephen Brown', *American Men & Women of Science: A Biographical Directory of Today's Leaders in Physical, Biological, and Related Sciences* (Detroit, MI: Gale, 2008), www.gale.com/uk/c/biography-in-context [accessed 4 July 2015]. For genetics at the NIDR see R. R. Harris, *Dental Science in a New Age: A History of the National Institute of Dental Research* (Rockville, MD: Montrose Press, 1989), pp. 273–5.
50 For the history of Cold War science see A. J. Wolfe, *Competing with the Soviets: Science, Technology, and the State in Cold War America* (Baltimore, MD: Johns Hopkins University Press, 2013). For biomedical sciences in particular see C. Hannaway and V. A. Harden, *Biomedicine in the Twentieth Century: Practices, Policies, and Politics* (Amsterdam: IOS Press, 2008); S. de Chadarevian, *Designs for Life: Molecular Biology after World War II* (Cambridge: Cambridge University Press, 2002).
51 M. M. Cohen, G. Cassady, and B. L. Hanna, 'A genetic study of hereditary renal dysfunction with associated nerve deafness', *American Journal of Human Genetics*, 13:4 (1961), 379–89.
52 R. Hudgins, 'Report of the research department, concerning heredity of deafness', *Clarke School Annual Report*, 95 (1962), 51–5; R. Hudgins, 'Report of the research department, concerning heredity of deafness', *Clarke School Annual Report*, 97 (1964), 39–41; R. Hudgins, 'Report of the research department, concerning heredity of deafness', *Clarke School Annual Report*, 99 (1966), 39–41.
53 For subtypes of genetic deafness and associated conditions identified throughout the 1960s see the seminal work of Bruce Konigsmark. B. Konigsmark, *Hereditary Deafness in Man* (White Plains, NY: National Foundation, March of Dimes, 1969).
54 For the development of biomedical computing see J. A. November, *Biomedical Computing: Digitizing Life in the United States* (Baltimore, MD: Johns Hopkins University Press, 2012), 67–89.
55 Anon., 'Chin Sik Chung', *American Men & Women of Science: A Biographical Directory of Today's Leaders in Physical, Biological, and Related Sciences* (Detroit, MI: Gale, 2008), www.gale.com/uk/c/biography-in-context [accessed 4 July 2015].
56 C. S. Chung, O. W. Robinson, and N. E. Morton, 'A note on deaf mutism', *Annals of Human Genetics*, 23 (1959), 357–66, here 357, 365.
57 C. S. Chung and K. S. Brown, 'Family studies of early childhood deafness ascertained through the Clarke School for the Deaf', *American Journal of Human Genetics*, 22:6 (1970), 630–44, here 643. Interestingly, the possibility of different populations having a different distribution and frequency of genes was not addressed much in this period.
58 Next to the studies already mentioned see e.g. P. J. Waardenburg, 'A new syndrome combining developmental anomalies of the eyelids, eyebrows and nose root with pigmentary defects of the iris and head hair and with congenital deafness',

American Journal of Human Genetics, 3:3 (1951), 195–253; L. S. Wildervanck, 'Hereditary malformations of the ear in three generations: marginal pits, preauricular appendages, malformations of the auricle and conductive deafness', *Acta Oto-Laryngologica*, 54 (1962), 1–6. For an overview of the nearly thirty syndromes known by the mid-1960s see L. J. Arthur, 'Some hereditary syndromes that include deafness', *Developmental Medicine and Child Neurology*, 7:4 (1966), 395–409.

59 National Institutes of Health, *Proceedings: Conference on the Collection of Statistics of Severe Hearing Impairments and Deafness in the United States, 1964* (Washington, DC: U.S. Government Printing Office, 1964), p. 8.

60 L. Fisch, 'Syndromes and early detection of deafness', *Reports of the Proceedings of the International Congress of the Deaf and the Forty-First Meeting of the Convention of American Instructors of the Deaf, Gallaudet College, Washington D.C. June 22–28 1963* (Washington, DC: U.S. Government Printing Office, 1964), pp. 627–32, here pp. 628, 630. Italics in original.

61 National Institutes of Health, *Proceedings, 1964*, pp. 13–14.

62 L. S. Wildervanck, 'The significance of associated anomalies in deafness', *Reports of the Proceedings of the International Congress of the Deaf, 1963*, pp. 632–8, here p. 638.

63 G. E. Shambaugh, 'Discussion: medical treatment and research', in F. McConnell and P. H. Ward (eds), *Deafness in Childhood* (Nashville, TN: Vanderbilt University Press, 1967), pp. 252–62, here 260.

64 *Clarke School Annual Report*, 100 (1967), 9.

65 William Ennis has recently argued that during the late nineteenth and first decades of the twentieth century, deaf people on average had a lower marriage rate and fewer children than the hearing population, and that eugenic reasons were a 'primary factor'. See Ennis, 'Hereditarian ideas', p. 21. While certainly eugenic reasons played a role, however, Ennis' basic assumption that deaf people's relatively low socioeconomic status should have led to a higher marriage rate and number of children would need to be accompanied by a more fine-grained analysis of various factors.

66 Chung and Brown, 'Family studies', 641.

67 See e.g. McConnell and Ward, *Deafness in Childhood*; F. H. Bess (ed.), *Childhood Deafness: Causation, Assessment, and Management* (New York: Grune & Stratton, 1977).

3

MINORITIES AND PATHOLOGIES: PSYCHOGENETIC COUNSELLING AT THE NEW YORK STATE PSYCHIATRIC INSTITUTE, 1955–1969

Are deaf people more or less likely to develop mental disorders, and if so, do they manifest differently than in a hearing person? What, in the first place, does their 'normal' mental and social life look like? These are questions that are still discussed today, often with the ableist assumption that hearing loss must result in psychosocial or intellectual deficiencies. The project explored in this chapter is often cited as a baseline, yet it is hardly ever taken in its full scope and ambivalence. From 1955 to 1969, an interdisciplinary research team under psychiatric geneticist Franz Kallmann explored these questions at the New York State Psychiatric Institute (NYSPI) Department of Medical Genetics. Their mental health project for deaf people established genetic and mental health care services that – for the first time in the US – considered deaf people a social minority who should receive care in their own, native sign language. Today, such health care services that consider the specific needs of linguistic or cultural minorities are relatively common in the US. Fifty years ago, however, this was a novelty, especially for a group that had long been denied this very sociolinguistic identity. Analysing these developments, this chapter ties the NYSPI mental health project to the post-war expansion of health services, community psychiatry, and a psychologization of both disability and genetic counselling that allowed for more relative definitions of deaf normalcy. Showing the complex transformation of public health-oriented eugenics into individualized genetics, it also makes visible how groups or individuals came to be defined as 'deviant', 'worthy', or 'defective'.

The project had explorative, applied, and collaborative dimensions. It resulted from a level of cooperation between the NYSPI and the New York State deaf community that was unusual for its time. On the explorative level, the NYSPI staff aimed to learn about the New York state deaf population and establish a baseline for what, in the first place, constituted mental health and illness in deaf people. When Kallmann and his colleagues began working with deaf patients and community members, they knew little about deafness. Rather than measuring deaf people by standards established for the hearing, they engaged in a large-scale survey of sociological, reproductive, psychiatric, and professional characteristics. On the applied level, the project established a wide range of psychiatric and social services, including a special inpatient unit for deaf patients at Rockland State Hospital, Orangeburg, NY, and a range of community and outpatient services, including support groups, family, and genetic counselling.

The last chapter traced the effect that the rapidly advancing, more sophisticated understanding of genetic deafness had on genetic counselling during the 1950 and 1960s. This chapter will focus on how, in the same period, but in a different context, deafness was redefined as a psychosocial condition, how deaf people came to be seen as a social minority – and why, surprisingly, psychiatric genetics was at the forefront of this development. With its claims that our emotions, sexual orientation, mental health and illness, in short, our fate and identity, are genetically predetermined, psychiatric genetics has acquired a reputation for disregarding sociocultural influences and perpetuating bias. Franz Kallmann, often dubbed the founding father of American psychiatric genetics, is a prime example of this reputation. Historians have usually portrayed him as a hard-line eugenic determinist at odds with the predominantly psychoanalytic psychiatric profession of mid-century America.[1]

Yet this is too simple a picture that does not do justice to the complexities of the interconnected histories of eugenics, genetics, disability, and the psychosciences. Indeed, Kallmann was a crucial figure in introducing psychotherapeutic motives to genetic counselling; an approach that also influenced the mental health project for the deaf. At the NSYPI, the goal of family and genetic counselling no longer was to prevent deafness per se, but to produce a happy, well-adjusted family and individual. The genetic counselling that established itself in the 1940s and 1950s was more individualistic and flexible than the heredity advice of previous decades. Historians have pointed out that it nevertheless perpetuated conservative family and gender roles. With its focus on middle-class respectability and on social adjustment, the NYSPI project, too, was rooted in the thinking of its time. It shows, however, that contemporary norms could morph and evolve when the target populations challenged them, and when professionals acknowledged their perspectives.

The previous chapters focused on institutions that treated deafness as part of the larger issue of childhood disability. This chapter focuses on professionals who worked with deaf adults and their organizations; a perspective that made a significant difference. The agency of children was always mediated by parents or institutional caregivers, such as teachers. For the NYSPI researchers, working with deaf adults from a similar middle-class background fostered exchange on a more equal level. As they began to engage and collaborate with the self-confident and well-organized New York State deaf community, their regard for deaf people grew, and their assumptions about deafness changed. Collaboration engendered a sense of identification, and blurred the line between professionals and that study population – not least because the number of deaf professionals in mental health and rehabilitation grew. As they got to know their deaf patients and research partners, deaf 'normalcy' came to mean something different to the NYSPI researchers than it had to professionals previously. Perhaps most importantly, they recognized deaf culture and community, and saw in deaf organizations important partners for collaboration.

Working with community members and deaf psychiatric patients, NYSPI researchers 'discovered' deaf people as a population in need of psychiatric services, yet neglected by professionals. The motives of neglect and professional remediation have a long tradition in the history of disability and deafness, usually accompanied by a strong dose of medical paternalism. Certainly, paternalism was present in the NYSPI project, too. Yet it also explored and established new forms of collaboration between professionals and the local deaf community. This collaboration between the NYSPI and local deaf communities unsettled established assumptions about deafness. It addressed the stigma of mental illness, and simultaneously reproduced hierarchies of difference: both sides could agree that being part of the deaf minority was a kind of 'normal', yet believed that mental illness was a condition that needed to be addressed, normalized, overcome, and prevented.

The project combined psychiatric and ethnosocial theories in a new form of minority services that would become highly influential. Within the next decade, other mental health centres for deaf people were established that followed the NYSPI model, for example in 1968 in San Francisco, and in 1969 in Chicago. The project also makes visible new ways of establishing professional authority, focusing less on fixing disability and more on equal access to health care services. Borrowing equally from Cold War rhetoric and the language of civil rights movements, NYSPI psychiatrists and geneticists portrayed themselves as experts who furthered democratic ideals by offering services to 'neglected' minorities. This made eugenic thought appear oddly compatible with minority activism.

Franz Kallmann: from sterilizing the 'feeble-minded' to counselling the deaf

Jewish-born, German-American Franz Kallmann remains one of the most controversial figures in the history of genetics and psychiatry. Depending on national and professional perspectives, portrayals range from highly esteemed founding father of psychiatric genetics to hard-core genetic determinist, almost a Nazi himself – a peculiar characterization for a scientist with a Jewish background.[2] Born in Silesia in 1897 to a Jewish family, Kallmann graduated from the University of Breslau in 1922 and began working as a neurologist and surgeon in a Breslau hospital. During this time, he converted to Protestantism, like many German Jews of his generation. Interested in neurology, psychiatry, criminology, and forensics, he continued his studies at the Charité hospital in Berlin, working under psychiatrist Karl Bonhoeffer and neuropathologist Hans-Gerhard Creutzfeldt. He also studied at the Berlin Psychoanalytic Institute, pursuing his lifelong interest in psychotherapy that would later inform his genetic counselling. In 1928, he became head of the neuropathological laboratory in the Berlin Herzberge Heil- und Pflegeanstalt. Here, he began to study the inheritance of schizophrenia. He systematically combed through hundreds of patient files, some of which dated back to the late nineteenth century, tabulating reproductive and hereditary patterns. His goal was to predict, and thus to prevent, the condition.[3]

In 1931, a research stay at the Deutsche Forschungsanstalt für Psychiatrie (German Psychiatric Research Institute, DFA) in Munich provided Kallmann with an opportunity to further pursue this interest. He worked with psychiatrist Ernst Rüdin, head of the DFA's influential Geneaologisch-Demographische Abteilung (Genealogical-Demographic Division, GDA), the first institution worldwide dedicated to the study of psychiatric genetics. Swiss-born Rüdin was one of the most influential figures in German psychiatry and eugenics. Using state-of-the-art statistical and demographic methods, he claimed to determine individual risk for mental disorders. His work and reputation attracted young scientists from Germany and abroad, many of them supported by Rockefeller Foundation fellowships. For this generation of upcoming psychiatrists – Kallmann among them – Rüdin's statistical approach linked individual diagnosis, public health, and wide-spread fears about degeneration. His students would later be influential in Germany and abroad. Franz Kallmann and Elliot Slater, for example, would found the first institutes of psychiatric genetics in the US and the UK respectively.[4]

Like his mentor Rüdin and many of his generation, Kallmann was concerned about the effect of supposed hereditary degeneration on public health.

As a preventative measure, he promoted sterilizing hereditarily 'defective' individuals, if necessary by coercion. He thus welcomed the 1933 Law for the Prevention of Genetically Diseased Offspring, passed shortly after the Nazis seized power. His research on schizophrenia as a recessive trait, he believed, would provide crucial input for applying the law. Thus, he proposed in 1935 to sterilize not only schizophrenic patients, but also family members, whom he believed carried a significantly increased risk for schizophrenia. Given this risk and the supposedly high occurrence of 'feeble-mindedness' in these families, he considered their offspring 'eugenically unwanted'.[5]

By Nazi definitions, however, Kallmann was Jewish, and thus unwanted himself. His hopes to continue working in Germany were soon shattered. Dismissed, without pay, from his position in 1935, he emigrated to the US in 1936 with Rüdin's support. In New York, influential anthropologist Franz Boas put him in contact with Nolan D. C. Lewis, head of the New York State Psychiatric Institute, who agreed to establish a small genetics division for Kallmann. The NYSPI was exceptionally well suited for a German emigrant who combined biogenetic psychiatry with psychoanalytic interests. Founded in 1895, and from 1929 located at the Washington Heights Columbia-Presbyterian Medical Center, the NYSPI emphasized biomedical research as a means to understand and cure mental illness. Over time, its departments came to include bacteriology, neuropathology, chemistry, biochemistry, neurochemistry, internal medicine, medical genetics, biological psychiatry, and behavioural physiology. Associated with Columbia University, it served as a research facility and training ground for residents at the Columbia School of Medicine.[6]

At first, Kallmann's genetics division was a one-man endeavour. After surviving some financial insecurity, however, it soon became a regular department. It was associated with Columbia University, where, from the mid-1940s to his death in 1965, Kallmann served as professor of psychiatry. Modelled after Rüdin's Munich GDA, his department was the first institute for psychiatric genetics and the second institute for human genetics in the US. Kallmann built his reputation in American genetics and psychiatry, publishing on twin studies, the heredity of mental illness or of homosexuality. He was a member of the American Eugenics Society; in 1948 he became a co-founder of the American Society of Human Genetics, and acted as its president in 1952. He was particularly well established in the New York State mental health care system. NYSPI director Nolan D. C. Lewis supported his work, as did Paul Hoch (who shared with Kallmann the experience of having to leave Germany as a Jew), president of the Society of Biological Psychiatry, who became New York State Commissioner of Mental Health in 1955.[7]

Kallmann's psychiatric genetics was not, as sometimes argued, an outlier in opposition to dominant psychoanalytic approaches in mid-century America. He was part of the psychiatric establishment, and his psychogenetics, imbued with psychosocial language, was attractive to a society simultaneously buoyed by post-war scientific optimism and paralysed by Cold War fears. Claiming to predict and prevent mental illness, psychogenetics allowed psychiatrists to cast themselves as the guardians of society's (mental) well-being. Kallmann, in particular, developed a vision of psychiatric genetics as a guiding science in 'a world of emotional unrest and rapid economic change'. It encouraged, he believed, responsibility for oneself and for society. Establishing the family as the 'indispensable biological, social, and educational unit', he promoted a message greatly appealing to pro-natalist post-war America with its idealization of middle-class family life.[8]

Historians have mainly focused on the continuities between Kallmann's work in Germany and the US, renouncing his self-portrayal as a morally upright scientist who had left Germany disgusted with 'the political abuse of genetics for racial purposes'.[9] Taking this first, German quarter of his career as the standard by which to measure him, however, overlooks the context of his thirty year-long career in the US, including his work with deaf patients and community members. This last project, encompassing the ten years from 1955 to his death in 1965, was the culmination of a lifetime's work in psychogenetics, eugenics, and preventive mental health. It was part of larger transformations from eugenic population studies to psychiatric genetics, from the mental hygiene movement to community psychiatry, and from legitimizing scientific interventions with improving populations to arguing with social justice, minority difference, and minority rights. On the local level, it was part of mid-century mental health reform in New York State that made possible collaborations between psychiatric genetics and minority psychiatry.

To help 'deaf people get more out of life, too': psychiatry as a service and consumer good

For American psychiatry, the 1950s to 1960s was an era of immense opportunity, expansion, and optimism. Located at the intersection of public health, biomedicine, and the social sciences, the field profited immensely from a steady expansion of federal funding in biomedicine and research. The National Mental Health Act of 1946 and the foundation of the National Institute of Mental Health in 1949 were the result of growing federal involvement in health care research and services. They provided the legal framework, and the financial, institutional, and professional resources to improve and expand research, training, and care, and to invest in the prevention of mental illness.[10]

A general, broad occupation with mental health drove this expansion. It concerned, first, the traditional clientele of psychiatry: patients in mental hospitals and asylums. Their situation in severely overcrowded and understaffed state hospitals became a matter of public debate after journalists and former patients publicly criticized inhumane conditions. De-institutionalization and establishing community mental health services were usually seen as the solutions to these problems, with mixed results over the coming decades. Yet increasingly, it was also the mental health of the ordinary citizen that came into the focus of psychiatrists and policy makers. Researchers found that enlisted men were affected by psychiatric conditions at an alarming rate; a finding considered a threat to the nation's ability to defend itself. Psychiatrists also anxiously observed civilians for signs of mental health disturbances caused by Cold War threats, and more generally by the stresses of modern life. Mental illness also increasingly was portrayed in movies, books, newspaper, and journals, enforcing the notion that mental health and emotional introspection were something for which every citizen should strive – and that mental health services were a consumer good to improve one's well-being.[11]

Community psychiatry, the guiding paradigm of post-war mental health care, aimed at all these groups. It was the effect of, and an answer to, the challenges of deinstitutionalization, of downsizing and improving conditions in overcrowded mental hospitals, but also of reaching patients with less severe mental health issues. Federal legislation enforced and encouraged the move towards community-based mental health care. The 1954 Community Mental Health Services Act, for example, aimed to prevent mental illness by investing in the improvement and availability of mental health services outside of the clinic. This political framework engendered multi-disciplinary projects, such as the one described in this chapter, with new professions previously not found in mental health care, for example (clinical) psychology or rehabilitation.[12]

New York State was at the forefront of these developments. With its enormous inpatient population – by 1945, the state's mental hospitals were overcrowded with 75,000 residents – and well-developed mental health administration, it was a spearhead in establishing community psychiatry and rehabilitation services. By 1940, the New York State Department of Mental Hygiene had established four aftercare clinics; by 1954, New York City operated several halfway houses that offered support for patients transitioning from hospital to the community.[13] This expansion of services and general occupation with mental health provide the backdrop without which the NYSPI mental health project for the deaf would not have been possible.

At first, however, deaf people did not seem to be included in the vision of psychiatric progress. Attending a 1950 psychology conference, psychologist Edna Levine observed that attention was on 'ways of helping people live fuller, happier lives'. Yet not 'one word', she noted with concern, 'was said about the deaf'.[14] Levine, who later called herself the 'god-mother of the project'[15] was familiar with both fields, psychology and deafness. She had begun her career as a teacher at the New York Lexington School for the Deaf before going on to earn a PhD in clinical psychology from New York State University in 1948, and dedicating her career to the psychology of deafness. This was a relatively new field. With very few exceptions (Fritz and Grace Moore Heider's work chronicled in Chapter 1), it was dominated by teachers with a pragmatic educational interest in testing and evaluation. Levine, too, had started her career as a teacher. But she also belonged to a new generation of professionals who turned the psychology of deafness into a distinct academic and professional field, a development made possible by the general growth of academic and rehabilitation psychology. What distinguished Levine and her colleagues from their predecessors was their involvement with the signing deaf community, and with the growing number of deaf professionals in rehabilitation and social service administration. Unlike most hearing professionals, and against dominant opinion, this younger generation of psychologists supported the use of sign language in deaf education, rehabilitation, and, more generally, in family and everyday life. In the early 1960s, Levine was a crucial figure in establishing the National Theater of the Deaf, which would perform in ASL. She brought together deaf and hearing actors and professionals and helped apply for federal grants.[16]

Levine's interaction with deaf professionals points to another important development. For a long time, deaf people had been excluded from entering the very professions supposed to serve them. In the 1950s, this was slowly but surely changing. During World War II and the post-war boom, opportunities opened up in administration, social services and (to a lesser degree) the sciences. Levine's colleague Boyce Williams was a pioneer in this regard. He was a key figure in improving services during his thirty-eight years as a consultant to the Rehabilitation Services Administration Programs for the Deaf, Hard of Hearing, and Speech Impaired.[17]

Like Levine, Williams was concerned about the lack of mental health care services for deaf people. Together, they began lobbying for a mental health centre in order to help 'deaf people get more out of life too'. Williams 'pledged his wholehearted support to this present pioneer endeavor'. They were able enlist the support of professional and deaf organizations. The attendees of the 1953 American Instructors of the Deaf meeting in Vancouver, for example, pledged to 'earnestly solicit the active assistance and encouragement of all interested organizations and individuals to the end that a Mental Hygiene clinic for the Deaf shall become a reality'.[18]

For Levine and Williams, like for many of their colleagues, psychiatric services were more than just a medical intervention for the small group of psychiatric inpatients. In an era of general prosperity and suburban growth, mental health services became a consumer good; and psychotherapy a popular tool for approaching the fears and frustrations of the ordinary citizen. Although it took white middle-class life as its norm, this expansion turned psychiatric services into a public good that was to be made available to the entire population. It was a means to achieve the 'good life' of post-war, consumerist, suburban America; something from which deaf people, like other minorities, were excluded, yet to which they were, in Williams' and Levine's opinion, entitled. This belief was essential for establishing minority services. Pointing to a history of neglect, it simultaneously offered a remedy.

Searching for a partner for realizing such mental health services, Levine contacted different New York institutions, including the NYSPI. There, she encountered Kallmann, 'who was also interested in the same goal' of improving mental health care.[19] It is unclear whether this was the first time he thought about working with deaf people, or, as Levine's wording suggests, he had come across deaf patients before in his extensive research in the New York State mental hospitals. Something about Levine's proposal, however, must have struck a chord with Kallmann, and engendered a mutual excitement for the project. As Levine recalled in a 1962 letter to him: 'I think back to our very first meeting and could fill pages with nostalgic "Do you remembers?" – all the iced tea that was consumed at the first meeting, the first patient we had, Mrs. Kallman's [sic] being the first to communicate manually, the marvellous things you did in securing State cooperation'.[20]

Enlisting Kallmann and the NYSPI ensured access to funding, staff, and resources. They secured, in 1955, a $27,800 Research and Demonstration Grant from the Office of Vocational Rehabilitation (OVR) for 'a mental hygiene clinic for deaf adolescents and adults'. The OVR, a press release explained, had taken an interest in improving mental health services in order to improve job training and placement records for 'emotionally disturbed deaf people'. In particular, the project was to address the 'inability of trained mental health workers to penetrate substantially the communication barrier of profound deafness'.[21] Support was renewed in 1963 for three more years in order to establish an inpatient unit for deaf patients, and in 1966 for another three years to initiate a range of preventive and rehabilitation services in various settings such as schools and support groups.[22]

In some ways, the mental health project for the deaf was the realization of Kallmann's professional vision: psychogenetics as an all-encompassing system that included family and genetic counselling, treatment, and prevention, all working towards the lofty goal of a society free from mental illness. The New York State deaf were to be the first population to which Kallmann hoped to apply such an all-encompassing system of mental health care. As he explained in 1962, their 'pilot study of family and mental health problems in a *deaf community* such as that of New York' served to 'illustrate the range and complexity of legitimate research and guidance functions which falls into the province of psychiatric genetics'.[23] Similarly, Kallmann's junior colleague John D. Rainer described the project as 'a psychiatric genetic department in action'.[24]

Yet the project was much more: it was a micro-laboratory that mirrored changes in psychiatric theory, treatment, and policies, and, not least, in patient and community involvement. Designed as a research and outreach programme in collaboration with the deaf community, it was to provide psychiatric services to a group of people long underserved and misunderstood by psychiatry. Staff members combined biological and psychosocial models of mental illness with pharmaceutical treatment, psychodynamic therapy, and psychosocial services. As a form of community psychiatry, it aimed to reintegrate individuals with mental illness into society. The project, Kallmann wrote, laid out 'a minimum action program for an aggregate of clearly frustrated but nonvociferous people who in an enlightened society would seem to need family guidance services with as much justification as any of their hearing counterparts'.[25] This rather paternalizing stance would weaken over the course of the project, not least as the staff discovered deaf people's metaphorical voice in a non-voiced language.

In 1955, project staff consisted only of Kallmann and two young psychiatrists, Columbia residents Kenneth Z. Altshuler and John D. Rainer. Like Kallmann, they had neither experience in working with deaf people, nor much knowledge of the existing literature and theories. Altshuler had come to the project by coincidence. After receiving a BA from Cornell in 1948 and an MD from the University of Buffalo in 1952, he was attracted to psychiatry because the field encompassed medicine as well as 'the study of the person'. After leaving the Navy in 1955, he continued his psychiatric residency programme at Columbia University. He was told to contact 'a man downstairs, named Franz Kallmann', who was 'starting a new project on working with the deaf'. Kallmann accepted him as a full-time researcher and resident while he completed his training in psychoanalysis. As Altshuler described their roles, Kallmann 'was the chief and there was another young doctor like me [Rainer], and ... we became the world's experts by default'.[26]

Soon, however, the project attracted collaborators from a wide range of disciplines. Over the years, staff grew to include more psychiatrists and psychologists, as well as educators, rehabilitation specialists, social workers, and other professions. Eminent statistician and management consultant W. Edwards Deming, widely known for popularizing the use of sampling techniques, helped with study design and data analysis; biological anthropologist Diane Sank, who would later work on the heredity of mental disorders, contributed to the analysis of family studies and genetic deafness. Next to Levine, who left in 1959 due to other obligations, another influential figure in the psychology of deafness joined the project: Austrian-born child psychiatrist Hilde Schlesinger (1925–2003), who in her long career published extensively on deafness and mental health, and in 1968 founded the University of California, San Francisco Center on Deafness. Like Levine, Schlesinger promoted the use of sign language, and thus helped steer the project to a trajectory different from the oralism still dominating professional approaches during the 1950s and 1960s.[27] Deaf professionals and community members, involved from the very beginning or joining later, likewise influenced this direction and encouraged a definition of deaf people as a social minority that was unusual for its time, but telling for things to come.

A 'world you will no doubt find strange': engaging with the New York State deaf community

By the 1950s, roughly a century of research had spoken about, but rarely with, deaf people. The NYSPI mental health project, on the other hand, had emerged as a collaborative enterprise between scientists and the deaf community. It had been initiated by a deaf professional – Boyce Williams – and, although most of the research staff was hearing, it signalled a willingness to engage in a more egalitarian manner. NYSPI researchers aligned themselves with a community of deaf adults, who they defined, by and large, as a functional social minority. In doing so, they justified their work with acceptance by and acquaintance with this community. Emphasizing the ideal of reciprocal partnership, staff members framed their professional roles not so much as one of fixing deafness, but as service-providers exploring or solving problems of social adjustment. This consumerist framework was not unproblematic, yet it resonated with deaf community leaders and individuals, and offered venues for contact and exchange.

The very attempt to provide some kind of accountability to and representation of the deaf community was highly unusual in mid-century America.[28] For deaf people engaged with the project this was a welcome change. Boyce

Williams lauded the project in 1958 as an example of progressive 'social action', contrasting it with the 'many places where nothing is done for the deaf'. He also conveyed a sense of ownership and influence when he remarked that 'to have the same services as the hearing would be one of our finest achievements'.[29]

Nevertheless, collaboration and exchange between professionals and the state's deaf community developed slowly. When the project first started, Altshuler recalled, 'the deaf got the impression that we were going to be treating them as special and imperfect'. However, 'once we explained that what we were trying to do was develop for them a parity of service, so that they had equal services with the rest of the state, they became very good friends of ours, and cooperated very well'.[30] In gaining the trust of community members and patients, the project had a significant advantage: from the very beginning, it had the explicit support of various deaf organizations. Community leaders from various organizations were represented on the supervising board, and important intermediaries liaised between the NYSPI and the deaf community. Edna Levine, for example, had long-standing ties with the New York deaf community; Boyce Williams straddled the line between expert and community member.

Conferences and workshops strengthened these ties and helped define necessary services. The first and largest of these bipartisan meetings was hosted by the NYSPI in June 1958, and included delegates from nearly forty deaf organizations. They represented national, state, and local organizations, including the National Fraternity Organization for the Deaf, the Empire State

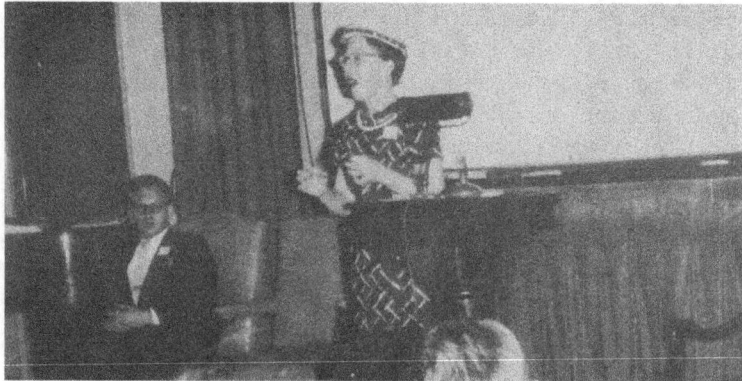

Figure 2 Edna Levine talking at a NYSPI meeting, New York State Psychiatric Institute, 1958 (reprinted with kind permission of the New York State Psychiatric Institute)

Association for the Deaf, the Bronx Silent Club, the local chapter of Gallaudet alumni, as well as religious organizations, e.g. the Hebrew Association for the Deaf. Unusual for the time, but in keeping with the NYSPI desire to foster communication and exchange, interpreters relayed from spoken English to sign language and vice versa.

Max Friedman, a 'specialist in vocational problems of the deaf' and a deaf member of the advisory council, gave the introductory speech. He did not shy away from criticizing the (hearing) NYSPI staff for being 'reticent in reporting its work to the deaf', and for leading 'too cloistered a life'. Then, addressing the deaf, he called for a heightened awareness of mental health issues. 'It is no disgrace', he asserted, 'to need the assistance of a mental health clinic, but it would be an everlasting disgrace if we deaf people, through false pride, should fail to support this most worthy project'. Such remarks provide some insight into the yet unwritten history of deaf people with mental illness. They address the shame and stigma associated with mental illness – yet also a willingness to address these issues.[31]

Ten years later, at a 1968 meeting titled *Psychiatry and the Deaf*, a panel of three deaf people presented their perspectives on 'Adjustment Problems of the Deaf' to psychiatrists and rehabilitation workers.[32] The three speakers represented a well-organized and vocal minority, whose achievements and deficits were seen as a matter of social disadvantage rather than inherent inability. Max Friedman once more portrayed himself as a self-confident partner for improving community services. He introduced his audience 'to a world you will no doubt find strange and to a people who badly need your services'. Psychiatrists, he pointed out, had been trained in the ways of the hearing rather than the deaf whose 'actions, thinking, and responses are apt to be unlike those of any other group'. He saw little wrong with these differences, and put the burden on the hearing, rather than the deaf: 'the communication problem is, to many of you, an insurmountable problem'. He welcomed the mental health project as a means to overcome a 'great shortage of psychiatrists who can work with the deaf', and offered the help of the myriad of New York State deaf organizations. They all, he assured, stood 'ready to be useful should you call on them for help or guidance'.[33] This collaborative spirit certainly was rooted in a sense of having, very recently, achieved progress in participation and recognition.

Friedman was followed by Naomi Leeds, president of the Mental Health Association of the Deaf. The Association had been founded in 1963 with the goal of raising awareness for mental illness in the deaf community and to support affected individuals moving from clinic to community.[34] It was not a patient organization. Rather, it had been established by Leeds and four more deaf New York housewives after they learned about the 'blight' of deaf patients in mental institutions.[35] The Mental Health Association of the Deaf was part of a larger trend for mental health and patient advocacy and activism that emerged in the 1960s and 1970s. Some activists and organizations challenged medical authority and severely criticized the oppressive nature of the mental health care system.[36] Others, however, like the deaf organizations in this chapter, took a more cooperative stance. They complemented professional with community services and shared with professionals the ideal of reintegrating recovering mentally ill patients into the community. Their work merits more attention, as does the perspective of mentally ill deaf people themselves, which, tellingly, has not yet been explored for this period.

Finally, Allen Sussman, the 'only deaf counselor in the Division of Vocational Rehabilitation in the State of New York' lamented the lack of professional opportunities and lingering discrimination that forced most deaf people to accept work below their education and abilities. Sussman later went on to a distinguished career in mental health and counselling, advocating for accessible mental health services for deaf people.[37] His career points to the limitations, but also to the opening of professional opportunities for deaf people. By the 1950s, a handful of individuals – among them Boyce Williams and Max Friedman – had broken through professional barriers and had achieved influential positions in public administration or vocational rehabilitation. Their number was rapidly growing, and here, too, the NYSPI project was pioneering. In research and clinical services, deaf staff members were considered a valuable asset and 'should be recruited or trained whenever possible'. The project also encouraged the involvement of 'educational and volunteer programs' such as the Mental Health Association of the Deaf as a supplemental support system.[38] Where previous research had painstakingly and paternalistically maintained the division between hearing expert and deaf object, the NYSPI staff signalled its willingness for cooperation and encouraged deaf people to enter a career in mental health care. From the initially sporadic contact with isolated deaf patients in mental hospitals, the project developed a model of active collaboration and mutual respect. Research and collaboration also set in motion a slow evolution in the perception of deafness and deaf people as a social and linguistic minority that in turn would influence mental health services.

Psychopathology and the 'normal' deaf adult: ambivalent results from an 'unknown' population

What engendered the unusual level of exchange and collaboration between NYSPI staff and local deaf communities? As Max Friedman had pointed out, deaf culture and sign language must have seemed new and foreign to the NYSPI researchers at first, although probably less so in New York than in less ethnically diverse locations. At the same time, there were also points of recognition. Certainly, shared middle-class values and assumptions between mental health professionals and deaf community leaders played an important role in finding common ground. Both sides embraced civic respectability and responsibility; values that deaf organizations had long upheld in their portrayal of deaf people as good, productive, and useful citizens. Their emphasis on responsibility and self-management resonated with mental health professionals, who promoted the ideal of the responsible and mindful citizen. Deaf organizations and NYSPI researchers thus shared an unspoken understanding of deaf people not as a deviant, but as a valued and under-appreciated minority. Certainly, this was a rather static and uniform definition of minority, which disregarded social, ethnic, and racial divisions and inequalities within the deaf community. Nevertheless, it was a perception of deaf difference that would have far-reaching consequences for research and services.

The fact that the NYSPI operated outside the established conventions of oralist surroundings and institutions played an important role. A sense of pioneering in an under-researched field permeated the project. As Kallmann recalled in 1962: 'the project began in something of a clinical and statistical vacuum'.[39] This was a telling statement. It ignored about half a century of psychological and educational research on deafness. Yet it also expressed a partial truth. Previous work had mainly focused on the intellectual development of deaf children in comparison to their hearing counterparts. The authors of these studies usually were (former) teachers, who often also served as school psychologists. Kallmann and his colleagues, on the other hand, worked primarily with psychiatric adult patients, and the deaf adult became their focus of research. This group indeed had been neglected in psychological and sociological research, with the exception of Fritz and Grace Moore Heider's research at the Clarke School. As Levine remarked in 1963, the deaf adult had remained 'a relatively unknown quantity in educational thinking'. Yet he or she 'most likely holds the key to many of the unsolved problems in the education of the deaf'.[40]

Staff members' self-portrayal as pioneers – or conversely their lack of grounding in previous research – signalled a willingness to start anew, and to discard old biases. Their excitement over mining 'an area so rich in theoretical and practical problems' merged with the ideal of helping 'a group so deserving and needy of psychiatric help ... so grossly neglected by our profession'.[41] The motives of benevolence and charity have been a constant in professional approaches to deafness, often tinged with a paternalism that talked about, but not with, service recipients. The NYSPI project in contrast explicitly addressed deaf people directly as valued collaborators in maintaining community mental health.

Setting themselves the task of delineating a normal range of behaviour, staff members were faced with finding standards of judgement. What, they asked, was it 'like to be a normal deaf person' – a question already pursued by Fritz and Grace Moore Heider in the 1940s.[42] Could something that was pathological in a hearing person be normal in a deaf individual? Unlike most previous research, NYSPI staff was willing to acknowledge that deaf people's differences in linguistic preference, behaviour, or reproductive patterns were not by definition deviant. At the same time, they struggled to define the attributes of a normal – socially well-adjusted and mentally healthy – deaf person. Studying the 'normal' deaf adult by example of the New York State deaf community thus was a means to better understand deviant or pathological behaviour. 'Unless one knows how the best adjusted members of a deaf group deal with such important personal matters as mate selection, marriage and parenthood', Rainer wrote in 1963, 'one cannot be constructive in attempting to help those who appear poorly adjusted'.[43]

In order to establish such a baseline of normal behaviour, the project engaged in a large-scale empirical study. Staff members sent out 8,200 questionnaires to all deaf residents of New York State over the age of twelve, of which 1,700 individuals replied; in 1958 they received a second questionnaire that focused on family structures, reproductive patterns and behaviour, age of onset of deafness, hearing status of parents, siblings and spouses, number of children, and age at marriage. Follow-up interviews with deaf people and their families, 'performed by psychologically trained research workers skilled in manual communication', further investigated education, vocation, and patterns of social interaction.[44] Twin studies provided a second set of data. Eventually, the study included a total of 110 twin pairs and two sets of triplets from New York State, New Jersey, Philadelphia, and Washington DC.[45] Certainly, this approach was shaped by Kallmann's empirical-statistic methods. Yet in contrast to his other work, it went beyond the question of genetics versus environment, and included psychological, cultural, linguistic, sociological, community, and patient perspectives.

The project's very definition of deafness, too, differed from previous approaches. For the NYSPI researchers, deafness was not so much an audiological-physiological as a psychosocial condition. Thus, it was defined in 1963 as a '*stress-producing hearing loss, from birth or early childhood, rendering a person incapable of effecting meaningful and substantial auditory contact with the environment*'.[46] Stress had become a leading explanatory category in psychiatry during and after World War II. Observing the aftermath of devastating battlefield experiences, psychiatrists emphasized environmental or social factors as the causes for mental illness and breakdown; and subscribed to the optimistic belief that removal of stress factors would restore mental balance. In deafness research, the emphasis on stress meant a shift from focusing on innate defects to emphasizing social and interpersonal factors such as bias and preconceptions.[47]

This new psychosocial definition of deafness also relied heavily on sensory deprivation research. Historian of science Mical Raz has traced the growing appeal of deprivation research, from laboratory experiments in the 1940s to an explanatory model for numerous social issues in the 1950s. Sensory deprivation was explored in the 1940s in experiments which temporarily disabled one or more senses, or isolated participants in dark, silent rooms for various periods of time. Exposed to such circumstances, participants displayed a variety of psychiatric disturbances. Conversely, in a form of circular reasoning, the fact that sensory deprivation could produce these disturbances was thought to provide insight to how and why they developed in first place. Soon, sensory deprivation research expanded into what became known as cultural and social deprivation. Impoverished environments, poor housing, or lack of social or intellectual stimulation in low-income and single-mother households were thought to deprive children of essential sociocultural stimuli and have devastating effects on their development. In their unquestioned reliance on white, middle-class norms, these studies were often highly biased. Yet they also pointed to the strong effect of environmental factors, and provided a hopeful narrative of potential social change if these environments were changed. There was also an explicitly political dimension in pointing to the devastating effects of neglect, discrimination, and impoverished environments. The motive of sociocultural deprivation became a staple in civil rights rhetoric, appearing, for example, in the speeches of Martin Luther King Jr.[48]

Temporary sensory deprivation in the lab was also thought to explain the experiences of people living with sensory differences; a problematic assumption. Deafness seemed to lend itself particularly well to the study of deprivation. Professionals had long been intrigued by the supposed effects of hearing loss on intellect and personality, yet only in the 1960s did they begin to explicitly apply the paradigm of deprivation. For psychologist Helmer Myklebust, for example, who in 1964 published one of the first monographs on the psychology of deafness, sensory deprivation was the key to understanding how deaf people functioned.[49] NYSPI researchers, too, evaluated the effects of sensoneural and psychosocial deprivation. Deprived of sound and speech, they theorized, deaf people had an inferior 'ability to conceptualize and synthesize ideas'.[50] Such statements went along with long-held preconceptions about deaf people's supposed lag in emotional and intellectual development and the belief that spoken language was necessary to develop abstract thoughts. Yet at the same time, NYSPI research also undermined these beliefs. Despite their 'developmental lacks and the omnipresent communication barrier', senior research psychologist George S. Baroff noted, deaf adults did not turn into 'withdrawn, isolated personalities'. On the contrary, they were able to 'establish adequate socialization patterns' and to 'participate in and utilize general community services'.[51]

Results thus were tauntingly ambivalent – and changed over time. In the beginning, NYSPI researchers had defined deafness as an innate disability that caused deficits and deprivations to which different people adapted with various degrees of success. With increasing collaboration and exchange, they came to portray deaf people as a stigmatized sociolinguistic minority group whose deficits were caused as much by maladjustment to and discrimination from majority society as by hearing loss per se. Overall, the researchers concluded, the New York deaf were a well-adjusted, content, and successful group. Indeed, they were a social minority with a 'unique subculture'.[52] This conclusion was not incompatible with defining deafness as a 'stress-producing condition' – the absence of hearing could contribute to the formation of a subculture – yet the values attached to each term differed. A stress-producing condition is something to be avoided or reversed; a subculture has an intrinsic value that researchers came to appreciate.

It might be unusual to locate the origins of such new, sociolinguistic, and relativizing definitions of deafness to a mid-century psychiatric research institution, much less to psychiatric genetics. But the NYSPI research was part of a larger trend of incorporating approaches from the social and psychosciences in exploring disability and difference. Certainly, these fields saw an unprecedented rise in influence in mid-century America, offering models for a vast range of phenomena, from family, gender, and parenting to racial relations or social unrest. Anthropologists tried to find universal human traits in cross-cultural comparison. Sociologists and psychologists focused on group dynamics to better understand bias, discrimination, and political orientation in the aftermath of Nazi Germany and fears of Communist subversion. Racial unrest and decolonization conflicts also fuelled psychosocial research, such as the work of Mauritian-born and Algeria-based psychiatrist Frantz Fanon. To activists in decolonizing countries and the West alike, Fanon's work provided a powerful model for understanding the situation of minorities in terms of oppressed identity and infantilizing disfranchisement.[53]

Interest in the sociology and psychology of minority groups opened the path for perceiving deaf people as such a group, too. In the 1954 *The Deaf and Their Problems* British teacher for the deaf Kenneth W. Hodgson commented for example: 'For the deaf themselves the real problem, of course, is not deafness but the fact of living in a hearing world'. 'Theirs', he continued, 'is a minority problem'. Such a portrayal turned deafness into a matter relative to one's social position rather than an innate disability. 'The deaf who lack natural speech are like foreigners in their own country', Hodgson stated. This similarity invited comparison with other minorities and even colonial power structures. 'In this country', he remarked for Great Britain, 'we have still a tendency to regard deafness as part of the White Man's Burden'. Instead of paternalistically doing 'things for the deaf because we are reluctant to realize how much they can do for themselves', he called upon their 'social self-reliance' as the only way to 'full citizenship'.[54] The NYSPI researchers came to a similar conclusion. 'Sociologically', project psychiatrists Arthur Falek and Michael Klaber explained in 1963, 'the deaf form a unique subculture, membership in which is determined solely by their physical disability'.[55] And Altshuler and Baroff theorized that deaf people experienced and had internalized 'minority group stereotypes' and feelings of inferiority.[56]

Such a psychosocial approach shifted blame and responsibility. Whereas before inferiority had been an innate fact of disability, now it was caused by inequality and bias. As Edna Levine specified: 'Having to grow up in a world of public ignorance and indifference, confused professional thinking, and untested professional hypotheses is the major handicap of early severe deafness'. Such a 'condition of psycho-educational malnutrition', she alleged, stemmed from the unfortunate, yet long standard 'proposition that the deaf child could be melded into a hearing one', if only he or she was treated as such. Here, deprivation theory became an instrument to criticize oralist ideals as an injustice committed against deaf people's natural rights and needs. Dismissing the rigid adherence to hearing normalcy that had dominated deaf education for so long, Levine advocated for exploring, accepting, and working with deaf children's difference.[57]

This sociopolitical perspective turned deafness into an extrinsic at least as much as an intrinsic disability: it was discrimination, prejudice, and ignorance from society that ostracized, excluded, and disadvantaged the deaf individual. Relativizing the dogma of normalization, this new paradigm legitimized minority difference within larger society. It depathologized deafness – and turned it into a political issue. Likening deaf people to other disadvantaged minorities such as African Americans, Hispanics, or immigrants turned their situation into an issue of social justice, denied rights, and missed chances. Thus, project psychologist Hilde Schlesinger argued in 1968 that deaf people's difficulties in education and social adjustment 'may be due not to deafness but to environmentally produced deprivation of those cultural factors shared by the middle-class American culture'.[58]

Like immigrant children, Schlesinger argued, deaf children lived 'within two cultures – the larger hearing America and the smaller deaf culture'. She pointed out that immigrant children who grew up bilingual and unashamed of their roots adapted more easily to US culture. They developed a self-confident trust in their own cultural standards, a 'healthy ethnocentrism', which was a prerequisite for normal intellectual and emotional growth. Deaf children were not so fortunate. Majority culture and misguided educational policies prevented them from developing such a healthy ethnocentrism. They experienced 'that one of their native tongues' – sign language – 'is not quite so good, not quite as acceptable, as the spoken language', even 'forbidden'. Social disapproval consequently created negative attitudes that inhibited the development of spoken language, too.[59] No longer a sign of backward pathology, sign language had become, on the contrary, a symbol of healthy childhood development, of comfort with one's physical and sociocultural self.

Attitudes towards sign language serve as a gauge for beliefs about deafness more generally. Sign language is a marker of difference; oralism signifies assimilation to hearing society. During the first half of the twentieth century, sign languages had been associated with primitivism, an ontological stage to be overcome on the path to civilization and citizenship. By the 1950s and 1960s, with a lessening of European ethnocentrism and changing standards of physical expressivity, public and professional sympathies shifted towards sign language and signing communities. Professionals began to show interest in sign languages. Ohio teacher for the deaf Benjamin M. Schowe Jr for example noted in 1958 that a growing number of people were 'studying the unsuppressible phenomenon of sign language'. He referred to the work of British linguist Sir Richard Paget, who had developed a system of manually coded English, and to Dutch linguist Bernard T. Tervoort, who studied the syntax of sign language in deaf children.[60] In the US, too, sign languages became the object of linguistic research. By far the most influential figure was linguist William Stokoe, widely credited with the 'discovery of American Sign Language as a true language'.[61] The notion of discovering an unknown language carried the (paternalistic) excitement of linguistic fieldwork in exotic locations, of bringing, as Stokoe put it in 1960, 'within the purview of linguistics a virtually unknown language'.[62] It is not surprising then that this re-evaluation of sign language coincided, as Douglas Baynton put it, with the 'reemergence of a romantic '"noble savage" image', that (once again) idealized sign languages as a natural language.[63]

Working with deaf people, the NSYPI staff, too, was confronted with the question of whether research, counselling, and therapy should be conducted only in spoken English or also in sign language. At first, Altshuler recalled, they tried to remain neutral in 'this running battle'. Yet practical considerations soon convinced them to use and learn sign language. Working with psychiatric patients, most of whom communicated manually, made relying on lip-reading and speech seem impractical, if not impossible. 'If you wanted to communicate with these folks', Altshuler elaborated, 'you had to know the language, and not knowing the language meant you were closed out of communication'.[64] Relying on interpreters was no solution. Interpreting by friends and family members was unadvisable in medical settings, and professional interpreting did not become widely available until the establishment of the National Registry of Interpreters for the Deaf in 1964. Moreover, interpretation introduced a potential source of miscommunication that might prove catastrophic in the assessment of psychiatric patients. Thus, in a time in which oralism still dominated education, and in which physicians expected their patients to communicate in spoken language, the NYSPI became the first institution to offer psychiatric and genetic services in sign language.

Sign language skills became mandatory for staff members, who attended weekly lessons. They were then assigned to deaf patients and had 'to learn on the job' – that is, in interaction with the patient.[65] In the spirit of mutual learning and collaboration, some of these classes were given by members of the local deaf community, including Max Friedman. A 1958 photograph shows him teaching sign language to staff members. The very composition of the photo reversed the established rhetoric of authority and expertise between deaf and hearing people. Demonstrating a sign, Friedman is standing at a lectern at the front of the room, towering over the sitting staff. They – young men and women in white coats – look up to him, smiling and observant. At the very back of the room, hidden by others and only visible at second glance, is Franz Kallmann, probably present for the photographer, but perhaps also learning some signs himself. This was radically new imagery, reversing the established order of things in which hearing experts relayed knowledge to deaf lay people.

Learning sign language soon proved to be rewarding. It was crucial for establishing a relationship with the New York State deaf community. Even making a 'little talk in stumbling sign language', Altshuler recalled, was highly appreciated, rare as it was in a time when most professionals working with deaf people had never even acquired basic signing skills.[66] Some knowledge of sign language also was indispensable in the clinic. When the project first looked for deaf patients in state hospitals, Rainer recalled in 1968, 'it was inspiring to us as well as to the patients, that, with our newly-acquired skills of manual

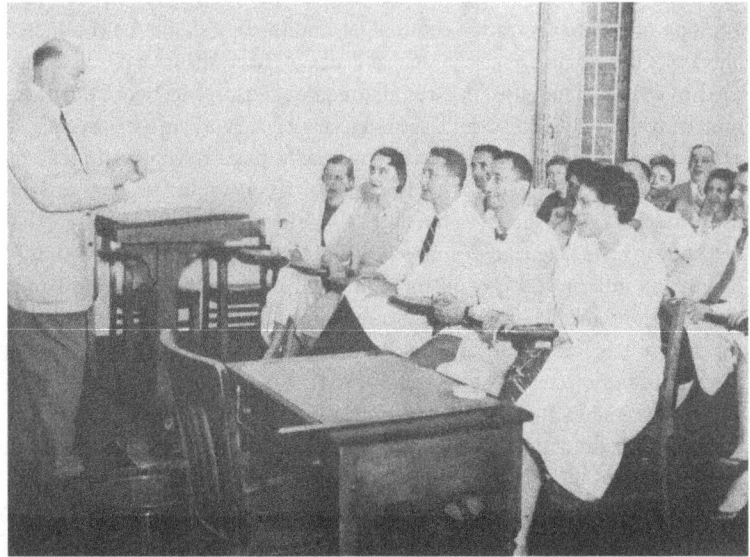

Figure 3 Project staff learning sign language, New York State Psychiatric Institute, 1958 (reprinted with kind permission of the New York State Psychiatric Institute)

communication, elementary as they were at the time, we were able to see the awakened contact, the chance to talk and listen, to persons who had not communicated with anyone in years'.[67]

New venues of communication allowed for new insight into deaf patients' behaviour, and questioned established stereotypes. Once psychiatrists engaged with them in their own language, the label of 'impulsive aggressive bizarre behavior' – a stereotypical diagnosis attached to deaf patients – turned out to be a chimera.[68] As Altshuler explained: 'we found, once we learned the sign language, that it wasn't always bizarre, it was based on some rationale, even if the rationale was a little whacko'. Establishing communication thus brought patients within the reach of contact, psychotherapy, medication, or vocational rehabilitation.[69]

This pragmatic embrace of sign language did not eradicate lingering preconceptions about its inferiority for expressing abstractions.[70] This meandering ambivalence characterized the entire project. Nevertheless, the basic assumption that deaf people required minority-specific norms and services guided psychiatric and genetic counselling.

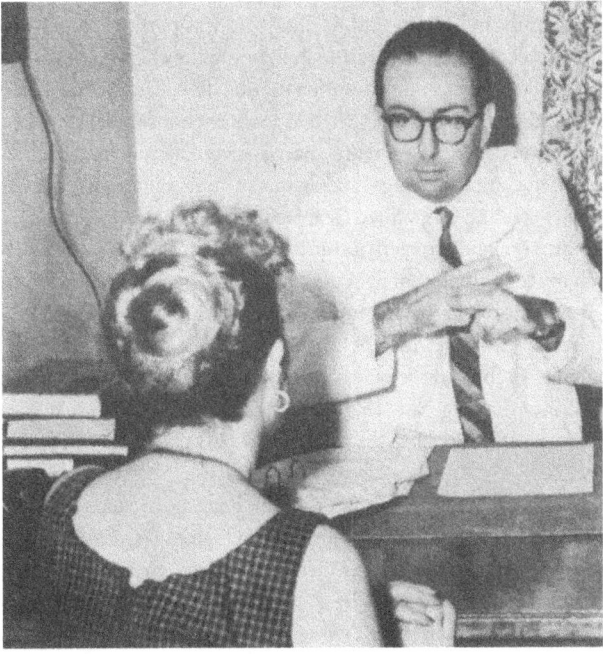

Figure 4 Psychiatric interview with a deaf patient, New York State Psychiatric Institute, 1958 (reprinted with kind permission of the New York State Psychiatric Institute)

'Prepared for family living in the fullest sense': eugenic goals and individual happiness

Family and genetic counselling was included in the range of psychiatric services offered by the NYSPI. In the early years of the project, staff members also contributed to the rapidly expanding research on genetic deafness. After Kallmann's death in 1965, however, pursuing basic research in the ever more complex field of biogenetics was beyond the staff's knowledge and capacities. Instead, Rainer, who succeeded Kallmann as project director and head of the NYSPI medical genetics department, Altshuler, and their collaborators focused on improving specialized services in family, psychiatric, and genetic counselling.[71] Unlike some of the psychiatric services, genetic counselling occurred in an outpatient setting with predominantly adult clients. They shared this outpatient setting with most medical and university institutions that offered genetic counselling in the 1950s and 1960s. At the NYSPI, however, family and genetic counselling also was part of a larger psychosocial research project that was interested in defining the characteristics of the target population. Their focus on preventing mental illness and social maladjustment rather than deafness itself changed the goals of counselling.

Explorations of deaf people's marriage and family patterns are a good example. Deaf intermarriage had been an area of much concern since at least the 1880s and Alexander Graham Bell's *Memoir*. Ever since, educators and researchers had worried about its potential dysgenic effect. The NYSPI researchers, too, noted that deaf people frequently married each other, yet for them, it was more of a fascinating than a harmful phenomenon. To Altshuler, intermarriage provided insight to the sociological factor of 'caste status ... associated with the various types of deafness'. From the psychiatrist's perspective, deaf intermarriage was less a genetic concern than a proxy for exploring sociological and psychological patterns, in particular, deaf people's status in society.[72]

Likewise, for Altshuler preference for hearing or deaf children was not reprehensible, but pointed to the need for genetic information. He noted that 'most persons from deaf families do not care one way or the other about the hearing status of their children'. Only 6.5 per cent of their study population preferred deaf offspring. Tellingly, it was not the preference for deaf or hearing children that perplexed Altshuler, but ignorance of how to achieve one or the other. 'Even among persons who prefer their children to be deaf', he exclaimed, 'there is no attempt to select the type of mate most likely to produce the desired result!'[73] Such an attitude appeared to him like lethargic ignorance towards realizing one's wishes (or at least towards learning about likely outcomes), when science and medicine could actually aid in their realization.

For the NYSPI staff, this 'pronounced lack of knowledge among the deaf about the workings of heredity' pointed to the dire need of making available 'specialized counseling services'.[74] Like many of his fellow geneticists Kallmann considered sex and marriage education instrumental for maintaining mental, social, and biological hygiene (or, in more modern terms, public and individual health). Thus, he lamented in 1963 about the 'remarkable dearth of information' at schools for the deaf 'about *genetically rooted family problems*'. Students' secluded upbringing in residential schools, he believed, contributed to their immaturity in matters of marriage and family planning. He advised that teachers should refer students to the nearest heredity clinic. Ideally, however, 'to be adequately prepared for family living in the fullest sense', students needed 'access at the proper time to special counseling programs'.[75] At conferences and in publications, Kallmann, Altshuler, Rainer,

Diane Sank, and other staff members promoted psychiatric genetics as the only field truly qualified for counselling the deaf on family, marriage, and reproduction. Careful to distance themselves from the coercive eugenics of the past, NYSPI researchers portrayed genetics as a rational, benevolent, and democratic science that countered misconceptions about heredity and enabled rather than restricted 'normal' family life. This focus on reproducing the 'normal' middle-class family was very much in keeping with the general image geneticists aimed to project in the 1950s and 1960s. Leading geneticists, who in the 1920s and 1930s had actively promoted coercive measures for the eugenically 'defective', now self-consciously focused on giving advice to a supposedly more rational group, namely ordinary middle-class citizens. When geneticist Sheldon Reed coined the term genetic counselling in 1947, he defined it as a non-directive service for the average couple or family wishing to establish a 'normal' family – that is, one without a disabled child. This focus on middle-class sensibilities also brought a shift towards incorporating the social and emotional dimensions of genetic knowledge and counselling. Reed considered genetic counselling a means to evoke and resolve parental feelings of fear, blame, and guilt. Kallmann, too, played an important role in defining genetic counselling as a psychosocial service that addressed and resolved client emotions in order to facilitate 'rational' reproductive decisions. Although it perpetuated contemporary family and gender norms, psychosocial and non-directive genetic counselling also allowed for more relative definitions of disability, dependent on client beliefs and expectation.[76]

At the NYSPI, this orientation towards the psychosocial benefits of counselling went hand in hand with a redefinition of deafness as mainly a psychosocial condition. Rather than preventing deafness per se, the goal of family and genetic counselling was to prevent the stress, maladjustment, and emotional disturbance it potentially caused. 'The most fruitful approach to prevention of maladjustment', explained Kallmann and Rainer in 1963, 'is to center attention on preparation for family living, since it is in this context that most unhappiness and behavior disorder manifest themselves'.[77] Kallmann's perspective as a psychiatric geneticist reveals the ableist bias inherent in this approach. 'It is tragic indeed', he remarked in 1953, 'to be married to a psychotic wife, or to have to send a schizophrenic son to a mental institution'.[78] As a psychiatrist, he considered mental illness far more damaging to the individual, family, and society than physical disability – a position that clearly influenced his research on deafness and psychiatry.[79] This hierarchy of disability and social worth mirrored – and still mirrors – general stigma in American society, where physical disability is considered a tragic fate to overcome and mental illness a frightening and uncontrollable loss of selfhood.

Counselling thus was a complex enterprise, whether it was a hearing man who wanted to marry a hearing woman with deaf parents, or a deaf person wishing to marry a hearing person. 'Counseling in such instances', Altshuler, Baroff, and Rainer advised, 'cannot be limited to estimates of the statistical risk of deafness in the couple's future children'. Rather, the counsellor had to 'take into account the emotional stability of the two persons involved and their attitude toward acquiring deaf relatives with the attendant possibility of social stigma'. The client's family and living situation was also evaluated, for example whether a hearing family felt comfortable with raising a deaf child or vice versa.[80] Such a multitude of hereditary, sociological, and psychological factors required an individualized approach. When it came to family planning, Rainer believed, 'the importance of considering each family on its own merits cannot be overemphasized'.[81] From the perspective of preventive mental health, the consequences of acquiring a deaf child, spouse, or relative thus were relational and relativistic: it was as much – or perhaps more so – a social issue, determined by attitudes, biases, and preferences, as a biological problem.

Given these multiple risks, psychosocial factors, and varied client backgrounds, the counsellor's role went beyond merely eliciting and evaluating facts. The 'qualified counselor', Kallmann wrote, needed to 'understand the given person's fears and hopes, defenses and rationalizations'. Ideally, 'sessions of this kind amount to explanatory or manipulative forms of *short-term psychotherapy* aimed at reducing anxiety and tension'.[82]

Falling into a time of intense debate over access to health care in the US, the NYSPI project also drew from a new sense of entitlement to medical services. Although wartime health services reached only part of the population, they raised expectations for such federal and state programmes to continue after the war. When, in 1944, President Roosevelt spoke about the right for universal access to health care, and when President Truman reaffirmed this vision in the late 1940s, they picked up on this shift in public opinion. Truman's proposal for universal health coverage eventually was defeated in 1950, yet the post-war era nevertheless saw an expansion of federal services in, and funding for, maternal health, childcare, rehabilitation, or mental health.[83] Social and minority activism also put public health and access to health care on their agenda: the peace movement worried about nuclear fallout and warfare, the women's movement linked political with reproductive rights, and Black activism tied community health to segregation, discrimination, and lack of resources. Often, these movements produced poignant criticism of the health inequalities inherent in and perpetuated by institutionalized science and medicine.[84]

It was exactly this combination of Cold War evocations of democracy and the ideals of minority health rights that allowed Kallmann and his colleagues to portray genetics as an integral service in a larger set of tools solving familial, health, or social problems. Rainer and Kallmann declared in 1963 that no 'group is more entitled to counseling for marriage, parenthood and genetics than the deaf'[85] – a phrase that geneticists would come to repeat in the following decades. Such language resonated with larger visions of equalizing access to health care for neglected populations. Vague as it was, this statement nevertheless evoked the ideals of a socially engaged psychiatry combating discrimination. It lent legitimacy to the project by claiming responsibility for deaf people as a group who had been denied access to basic services.

If one argued for the general benevolence of psychogenetics for individual and family, expanding its reach to 'underserved' minorities was only logical and inevitable. To question this expansion was to support discrimination against deaf people, and was therefore implicitly undemocratic. This line of thought turned genetic knowledge into a crucial form of self-knowledge, a prerequisite for a fulfilled life as an equal in a still unequal society. Conversely, to be an enlightened, rational citizen meant acting according to the principles of modern science.

Kallmann's justification of psychogenetics as a matter of rights and services points to an important shift in portraying the targets of eugenic improvement. Like most eugenicists during the early decades of the twentieth century, he had been an ardent proponent of coercive sterilization. By the 1950s, however, such coercive measures had fallen out of favour (though not necessarily out of practice). Attention shifted from the 'feeble-minded' and 'defective' to the more or less average citizen and family. Now, the reasoned expert upheld the ideal of eugenic responsibility towards oneself and society. 'In a democratic society, which rejects compulsory methods of public health planning', Kallmann wrote in 1953, 'it would seem a mandatory obligation for public health authorities to make adequate provision for expert guidance on problems of marriage, parenthood, and inheritance where it is needed and sought voluntarily by morally responsible people'.[86] Whereas the 'defective' and 'feeble-minded' had been treated as quasi-offenders, persecuted for endangering public health, Kallmann's new objects of research, deaf people, came to be defined as an oppressed minority group, who had been denied access to their basic right to psychogenetic services.

Historians have pointed out that such democratic rhetoric often merely veiled older eugenic beliefs and bias. Indeed, eugenic goals and thought remained omnipresent in talking about disability in mid-century America and beyond. The NYSPI project was no exception, yet it also makes visible important changes in beliefs about disability, professional authority, and client autonomy. In part, this was a generational shift, observable in the cooperation between Kallmann, the German emigrant born in the 1890s, and his American collaborators, who began their careers in the 1950s. Working with Kallmann, Altshuler and Rainer had come to embrace psychogenetics as crucial for modern psychiatry. Like their mentor, they considered genetic awareness a pillar of preventative mental health. Their opinions differed from his, however, when it came to the goals of counselling and the authority of the counsellor. For decades, Kallmann pursued psychogenetics with the vision of eventually ridding society of mental illness – a goal that required individual sacrifices. Although by the 1960s he no longer supported coercive sterilization, he continued to advise that couples with a family history of mental illness should refrain from having children of their own.

For Altshuler and Rainer, on the other hand, the individual's psychological and emotional concerns and preferences took precedence over eugenic population improvement. 'While it is unlikely that deafness or mental illness will disappear through such eugenic measures', they wrote in 1966 in reference to their genetic services, 'the relief of anxiety or avoidance of certain tragedy of even a single person cannot be overvalued'.[87] For them, reproductive decisions were the matter of the informed patient. When, in a 1968 workshop, a participant asked whether the project aimed 'to control deafness as a genetic factor', Altshuler's reply remained ambivalent. He pointed to the lack of definite knowledge on the inheritance of deafness in individual clients, which made advice difficult. In the spirit of non-directive counselling, he emphasized that staff did 'not attempt to influence their choice of marriage partners. We believe that they are entitled to make their choice on the basis of as much information as possible and full awareness of what is likely to ensue'.[88]

Conclusion

At first glance, Franz Kallmann and his NYSPI Department of Medical Genetics may seem like an unexpected location for a paradigmatic shift towards a more sociocultural model of deafness, and for a more relative, psychosocial approach to genetic counselling. Kallmann is often considered an example for the long-lasting influence of deterministic, anti-individualistic eugenics. Some scholars continue to criticize his hereditary determinism and stigmatizing view of minorities. Sociologist Graham Kinloch, for example, referred to his schizophrenia research as an example of 'extremely negative' majority attitudes towards deviants 'defined as psychologically and genetically defective'.[89] Ironically, others have lauded his work with deaf people as an example for minority-specific genetic and psychiatric services.[90]

The NYSPI mental health project for the deaf does not dissolve these contradictions, but makes visible ambivalent developments. Post-war genetics continued to perpetuate conservative social and gender norms, albeit behind a more liberal façade. Adherence to social norms remained important for NYSPI psychiatrists, too, yet the norms to be achieved changed and became more flexible. As long as deaf clients moved within the norms of middle-class respectability and sexuality, the question was not primarily how to eradicate or prevent deafness, but how to adapt psychiatric services, so that deaf people, too, could profit. This would become an important theme in genetic counselling for deafness in the following decades.

More generally speaking, such shifting perceptions of normalcy and pathology allowed fruitful collaborations with some, but not all groups or minorities. While Kallmann came to acknowledge deaf people as a valuable social minority, he continued to define homosexuality as a genetically determined social deviance; a definition that perpetuated harmful stereotypes and played into the larger crackdown on homosexual men in the 1950s 'lavender scare'.[91] The NYSPI mental health project was one among many reform projects in post-war psychiatry and rehabilitation that introduced new forms of cooperation and contact between professionals and target groups. It was based on a mutual understanding between professionals (the majority hearing, some deaf) and deaf community leaders: both sides believed that deaf people had been neglected in psychiatric care, and that it was time for professionals and the deaf community to make up for this neglect. Community psychiatry required that psychiatrists engaged with and got to know their target population, and even turn them into mental health care professionals themselves. This collaboration, however, was based on a narrow and static definition of community and minority. It was rooted in a notion of white middle-class respectability shared both by project staff and community leaders, muting social, ethnic, and racial divisions, and inequalities within the deaf community.

In sum, the NYSPI project influenced genetic deafness research and counselling in three ways: first, the collaboration with the New York State deaf community was crucial for these shifting perceptions of deaf people. There were certainly remnants of medical paternalism, yet the ideal of collaboration with patients and target communities left room for more diverse and less pathological perspectives. Unlike previous research, the NYSPI's community model was built on the contribution of deaf community leaders, members, patients, and, not least, a growing number of deaf activists. In this process, deaf people came to be defined as a minority with its own culture and language, who faced discrimination and bias from society at large, yet, overall, was well adjusted. This notion of countering supposed neglect with tailor-made services foreshadowed later projects that considered hearing loss the uniting factor of their target population rather than the pathological trait to target. At the same time, staff believed that the intrinsic and extrinsic factors of living with deafness put deaf people at a particular risk for emotional stress and maladjustment. Counselling thus required a comprehensive appraisal of individual life situations as well as an awareness of specific socio-psychological issues. Genetic counselling fashioned itself as a form of support and 'short-term' therapy, thus turning genetics into an essential form of self-knowledge. The importance of genetic awareness thus went beyond matters of reproduction. It was a matter of achieving a happy, fulfilled life as an equal citizen.

Second, the NYSPI project introduced the logic and rhetoric of minority-specific counselling. It was a forerunner for psychiatric and genetic services that justified specialized services with a 'neglected' minority's right to adequate health care in their own language. Vice versa, the language of minority rights and discrimination became entwined with professional self-portrayals. Here, we can see how ideologically loaded terms like democracy and discrimination, minority, and culture came to be used to justify medical or scientific interventions, and to establish forms of identity based on the confluence of science and social activism.

Third, the NYSPI project established a professional cluster of psychiatrists, psychologists, rehabilitation workers, and geneticists who acknowledged, accepted, or even embraced deaf culture and community. Working with adults, their approach differed significantly from the oralist-curative model that was the focus of previous chapters, and that continued to dominate most branches of science and medicine. In the remaining two chapters, we will see how this gap between different professional approaches to deafness would grow ever wider, as some geneticists came to identify with the demands of disability and Deaf movements.

Notes

1 For Kallmann see e.g. F. Mildenberger, 'Auf der Spur des "scientific pursuit": Franz Josef Kallmann (1897–1965) und die rassenhygienische Forschung', *Medizinhistorisches Journal*, 37:2 (2002), 183–200; A. Cottebrune, 'Franz Josef Kallmann (1897–1965) und der Transfer psychiatrisch-genetischer Wissenschaftskonzepte vom NS-Deutschland in die U.S.A', *Medizinhistorisches Journal*, 44:3–4 (2009), 296–324; V. Roelcke, 'Die Etablierung der psychiatrischen Genetik in Deutschland, Grossbritannien und den USA, ca. 1910-1960: zur untrenn-

baren Geschichte von Eugenik und Humangenetik', *Vorträge und Abhandlungen Zur Wissenschaftsgeschichte* (2002/2003 and 2003/2004), 173-90; V. Roelcke, 'Eugenic concerns, scientific practices: international relations and national adaptations in the establishment of psychiatric genetics in Germany, Britain, the USA, and Scandinavia 1910-1960', in B. M. Felder and P. Weindling (eds), *Baltic Eugenics: Bio-Politics, Race and Nation in Interwar Estonia, Latvia and Lithuania 1918-1940* (Amsterdam: Rodopi, 2013), pp. 301-33. For Kallmann's role in introducing psychotherapeutic thought into genetic counselling see Schmidt, 'Birth defects'.

2 For this characterization see e.g. R. C. Lewontin, S. P. R. Rose, and L. J. Kamin, *Not in Our Genes: Biology, Ideology, and Human Nature* (New York: Pantheon Books, 1984), pp. 207-9.

3 B. Glass, 'In memoriam, Franz J. Kallmann', *Proceedings of the Annual Meeting of the American Psychopathological Association*, 55 (1967), 322-32. For Kallmann's conversion to Protestantism, I follow Mildenberger who had access to his personal papers and correspondence. See Mildenberger, 'Auf der Spur des "scientific pursuit"', 185-6.

4 See Roelcke, 'Die Etablierung der psychiatrischen Genetik in Deutschland', 177-8, 184-7; Mildenberger, 'Auf der Spur des "scientific pursuit"', 186-7.

5 'eugenisch unerwünscher Nachwuchs' in the original. See F. J. Kallmann, 'Die Fruchtbarkeit der Schizophrenen', in H. Harmsen (ed.), *Bevölkerungsfragen: Bericht d. Internat. Kongresses f. Bevölkerungswissenschaft, Berlin, 26. Aug.-1. Sept. 1935* (Munich: J. F. Lehmanns Verlag, 1936), pp. 725-9, here p. 728.

6 Mildenberger, 'Auf der Spur des "scientific pursuit"', 184-8; Roelcke, 'Die Etablierung der psychiatrischen Genetik in Deutschland', 185. For the NYSPI see L. C. Kolb and L. Roizin, *The First Psychiatric Institute: How Research and Education Changed Practice* (Washington, DC: American Psychiatric Press, Inc., 1993), pp. 99, 104, 109-10, 129.

7 Roelcke, 'Die Etablierung der psychiatrischen Genetik in Deutschland', 186; Mildenberger, 'Auf der Spur des "scientific pursuit"', 188-92; Kolb and Roizin, *Institute*, pp. 17, 76, 82. For the history of medical genetics at the NYSPI see L. Erlenmeyer-Kimling, 'Medical genetics', in B. A. Fallon, J. M. Gorman, J. M. Oldham, and H. Pardes (eds), *The New York State Psychiatric Institute: American Psychiatry at the Centennial 1896-1996* (New York: The New York State Psychiatric Institute, 1998), pp. 33-42.

8 F. J. Kallmann, *Heredity in Health and Mental Disorder: Principles of Psychiatric Genetics in the Light of Comparative Twin Studies* (New York: Norton, 1953), p. 276.

9 J. D. Rainer, 'The contributions of Franz Josef Kallmann to the genetics of schizophrenia', *Behavioral Science*, 11:6 (1955), 413-37, here 414.

10 See G. N. Grob, *From Asylum to Community: Mental Health Policy in Modern America* (Princeton, NJ: Princeton University Press, 1992), pp. 5-7, 45-65; G. N. Grob, 'Creation of the National Institute of Mental Health', *Public Health Reports*, 111:4 (1996), 378-81.

11 For these developments see e.g. M. Halliwell, *Therapeutic Revolutions: Medicine, Psychiatry, and American Culture, 1945–1970* (New Brunswick, NJ: Rutgers University Press, 2014), pp. 17–47; H. Pols, 'War neurosis, adjustment problems in veterans, and an ill nation: the disciplinary project of American psychiatry during and after World War II', in G. Eghigian, A. Killen, and C. Leuenberger (eds), *The Self as Project: Politics and the Human Sciences* (Chicago, IL: University of Chicago Press, 2007), pp. 72–92; R. W. Schoeberlein, '"Maryland's shame": photojournalism and mental health reform, 1935–1949', *Maryland Historical Magazine*, 98:1 (2003), 34–72.
12 See Grob, 'Creation of the National Institute'.
13 See B. Weddle, *Mental Health in New York State, 1945–1998: A Historical Overview* (Albany, NY: The Archives, 2000).
14 Gallaudet University Archives, Manuscript Collection, MSS 166, Levine, Edna Simon, Box 21, Folder 31, 'Speeches, Mental Health Center for the Deaf', April 1958, p. 1.
15 Gallaudet University Archives, Manuscript Collection, Box 5, Folder 49, correspondence Kallmann Franz J., 'Levine to Kallmann', 17 December 1962.
16 For Levine see Anon., 'Edna Simon Levine', *Contemporary Authors Online* (Detroit, MI: Gale, 2008), www.gale.com/uk/c/biography-in-context [accessed 4 July 2015]; Gallaudet University Archives, Manuscript Collection, MSS 166, 'Biographical Sketch, Edna Simon Levine'. For the National Theater of the Deaf and Levine's role see S. C. Baldwin, *Pictures in the Air: The Story of the National Theatre of the Deaf* (Washington, DC: Galludet University Press, 1998), pp. 6–17.
17 For Williams see A. V. Thomkins, 'Williams, Boyce R (1910–1998), advocate for deaf people, federal government official', in S. Burch, *Encyclopedia of American Disability History: Vol. 3* (New York: Facts On File, 2009), pp. 969–70.
18 Gallaudet University Archives, Manuscript Collection, MSS 166, Box 15, Folder 22, draft proposal, undated [c. 1953] 'Mental Health project for the deaf, objectives and progress reports', p. 2.
19 Gallaudet University Archives, MSS 166, Levine, Edna Simon, Box 21, Folder 31, April 1958, 'Speeches, Mental Health Center for the Deaf', p. 2.
20 Gallaudet University Archives, Manuscript Collection, Box 5, Folder 49, correspondence Kallmann Franz J., 'Levine to Kallmann', 17 December 1962.
21 Gallaudet University Archives, MSS 166, Levine, Edna Simon Box 4, Folder 14, Correspondence Department of Health, Education and Welfare, 'OVR Press release', 25 March 1955, p. 1.
22 See J. D. Rainer and K. Z. Altshuler, *Psychiatry and the Deaf: Workshop for Psychiatrists on Extending Mental Health Services to the Deaf* (Washington, DC: U.S. Department of Health, Education, and Welfare, Social and Rehabilitation Service, 1968); J. D. Rainer and K. Z. Altshuler, *Expanded Mental Health Care for the Deaf: Rehabilitation and Prevention* (Washington, DC.: U.S. Department of Health, Education, and Welfare, Rehabilitation Services Administration, 1971).
23 F. J. Kallmann, 'Genetic research and counseling in the mental health field, present

and future' in F. J. Kallmann, L. Erlenmeyer-Kimling, E. V. Glanville, and J. D. Rainer (eds), *Expanding Goals of Genetics in Psychiatry: Anniversary Symposium of the Department of Medical Genetics, New York State Psychiatric Institute, October 27–28, 1961* (New York: Grune & Stratton, 1962), pp. 250–5, here p. 253. Emphasis in original.
24 Rainer, 'The contributions of Franz Josef Kallmann', 428.
25 Kallmann, 'Genetic research', p. 253.
26 'Oral history interview with Kenneth Z. Altshuler', Dallas/Baltimore, 6 February 2014, Interviewer: Marion Schmidt.
27 J. H. Zamora, 'Hilde Schlesinger – UCSF Doctor, Deaf Advocate', *SF Gate* (October 7 2003).
28 Grob, *Asylum*, pp. 125–72; For the growing involvement of other disciplines in psychiatry see J. G. Kelly, 'The National Institute of Mental Health and the founding of the field of community psychology', in W. E. Pickren and S. F. Schneider, *Psychology and the National Institute of Mental Health: A Historical Analysis of Science, Practice, and Policy* (Washington, DC: American Psychological Association, 2005), pp. 233–60.
29 B. Williams, 'Salutatory statement', in J. D. Rainer (ed.), *Mental Health Planning for the Deaf, Report of a Conference of New York State Organizations for the Deaf, held at the New York State Psychiatric Institute on June 14, 1958* (New York, 1958), p. 205.
30 'Oral history interview with Kenneth Z. Altshuler'.
31 Rainer, *Mental Health Planning*, pp. 11–12.
32 F. Friedman, N. Leeds, and A. Sussman, 'Adjustment problems of the deaf: panel of deaf adults', in Rainer and Altshuler (eds), *Psychiatry and the Deaf*, pp. 25–36.
33 *Ibid.*, p. 29.
34 *Ibid.*, p. 31.
35 While the association does not seem to exist anymore, it was active into the 1980s. See the Empire State Association for the Deaf Collection at the Rochester Institute of Technology Archives, which also contain programmes for plays and community activities.
36 N. Tomes, 'From outsiders to insiders: the consumer-survivor movement and its impact on U.S. mental health policy', in B. Hoffman, N. Tomes, R. Grob, and M. Schlesinger (eds), *Patients as Policy Actors* (New Brunswick, NJ: Rutgers University Press, 2011), pp. 112–31.
37 'Adjustment problems', p. 33. For Sussman's work and career in counselling see e.g. A. E. Sussman and L. G. Stewart, *Counseling with Deaf People* (New York: Deafness Research and Training Center, New York University School of Education, [1971] 1988).
38 Rainer and Altshuler, *Expanded Mental Health Care*, pp. iii–iv.
39 Kallmann, 'Genetic research', p. 253.
40 E. Levine, 'Historical review', in J. D. Rainer, K. Z. Altshuler, and F. J. Kallmann, *Family and Mental Health Problems in a Deaf Population* (New York: New York State Psychiatric Unit, 1963), pp. xvii–xxvi, here pp. xxv, xxvi.

41 J. D. Rainer, 'Background and history of New York State mental health program for the deaf', in Rainer and Altshuler (eds), *Psychiatry and the Deaf*, pp. 1–4, here p. 2.
42 'Oral history interview with Kenneth Z. Altshuler'.
43 J. D. Rainer, 'Introduction', in Rainer, Altshuler, and Kallmann (eds), *Family and Mental Health*, p. xiii.
44 K. Z. Altshuler, 'Sexual patterns and relationships', in Rainer, Altshuler, and Kallmann (eds), *Family and Mental Health*, pp. 92–112, here p. 92.
45 D. Sank, 'Genetic aspects of early total deafness', in Rainer, Altshuler, and Kallmann (eds), *Family and Mental Health*, pp. 28–81, here pp. 31, 46.
46 Rainer, 'Introduction', p. xiv, italics in original.
47 See e.g. T. M. Brown, '"Stress" in US wartime psychiatry: World War II and the immediate aftermath', in D. Cantor (ed.), *Stress, Shock, and Adaptation in the Twentieth Century* (Rochester, NY: University of Rochester Press, 2014), pp. 121–41; E. Ramsden, 'Stress in the city: mental health, urban planning, and the social sciences in the postwar United States', in Cantor (ed.), *Stress*, pp. 291–319.
48 M. Raz, 'Was cultural deprivation in fact sensory deprivation? Deprivation, retardation and intervention in the USA', *History of the Human Sciences*, 24:1 (2011), 51–69; M. Raz, 'The deprivation riots: psychiatry as politics in the 1960s', *Harvard Review of Psychiatry*, 21:6 (2013), 345–50.
49 H. R. Myklebust, *The Psychology of Deafness: Sensory Deprivation, Learning, and Adjustment* (New York: Grune & Stratton, 1964).
50 M. Klaber and A. Falek, 'Delinquency and crime', in Rainer, Altshuler, and Kallmann (eds), *Family and Mental Health*, pp. 141–51, here pp. 147–9.
51 G. S. Baroff, 'Patterns of socialization and community integration', in Rainer, Altshuler, and Kallmann (eds), *Family and Mental Health*, pp. 113–15, here pp. 113, 115.
52 Klaber and Falek, 'Delinquency', p. 143.
53 For anthropology see T. Teslow, *Constructing Race: The Science of Bodies and Cultures in American Anthropology* (New York: Cambridge University Press, 2014). In the social sciences, Adorno's, Sanford's and Brunswick's 1950 study of the authoritarian personality became highly influential. See T. W. Adorno, E. Frenkel-Brunswik, D. J. Levinson, and N. Sanford, *The Authoritarian Personality* (New York: Harper, 1950). For Fanon see e.g. J. McCulloch, *Black Soul, White Artifact: Fanon's Clinical Psychology and Social Theory* (Cambridge: Cambridge University Press, 1983).
54 K. W. Hodgson, *The Deaf and Their Problems: A Study in Special Education* (New York: Philosophical Library, 1954), pp. 347, 355.
55 Klaber and Falek, 'Delinquency', p. 143.
56 K. Z. Altshuler and G. S. Baroff, 'Educational background and vocational adjustment', in Rainer, Altshuler, and Kallmann (eds), *Family and Mental Health*, pp. 116–30, here p. 127.
57 Levine, 'Historical review', pp. xvii–xxvi, xxvi.
58 H. Schlesinger, 'Cultural and environmental influences in the emotional devel-

opment of the deaf', in Rainer and Altshuler (eds), *Psychiatry and the Deaf*, pp. 128–31, here p. 128.
59 *Ibid.*, pp. 128–31.
60 B. M. Schowe, 'Some observations on sign language', *Educational Research Bulletin*, 37:5 (1958), 120–4, here 120, 122.
61 J. R. Gannon, J. Butler, and L.-J. Gilbert, *Deaf Heritage: A Narrative History of Deaf America* (Silver Spring, MD: National Association of the Deaf, 1981), p. 364.
62 W. C. Stokoe, *Sign Language Structure: An Outline of the Visual Communication Systems of the American Deaf* (Buffalo, NY: Department of Anthropology and Linguistics, University of Buffalo, 1960) pp. 3, 67.
63 Baynton, *Forbidden Signs*, p. 156.
64 'Oral history interview with Kenneth Z. Altshuler'.
65 *Ibid.*
66 *Ibid.*
67 Rainer, 'Background', p. 2.
68 'Oral history interview with Kenneth Z. Altshuler'.
69 *Ibid.*
70 See e.g. R. R. Grinker, 'Conference summary and comments', in Rainer and Altshuler (eds), *Psychiatry and the Deaf*, pp. 147–53, here p. 152.
71 See J. D. Rainer and W. E. Deming, 'Demographic aspects: number, distribution, marriage and fertility statistics', in Rainer, Altshuler, and Kallmann (eds), *Family and Mental Health*, pp. 13–27.
72 Altshuler, 'Sexual patterns and relationships', pp. 99, 107, 108.
73 *Ibid.*, p. 108.
74 *Ibid.*, p. 107.
75 F. J. Kallmann, 'Some genetic aspects of deafness and their implications for family counseling', in *Reports of the Proceedings of the International Congress of the Deaf*, 1963, pp. 639–62, here pp. 639, 642. Italics in original.
76 For the history of non-directive counselling and the incorporation of psychosocial motives see e.g. Ladd-Taylor, '"A kind of genetic social work"'; Stern, *Telling Genes*; Paul, *Controlling Human Heredity*, pp. 125–7. For Kallmann's role in particular see Schmidt, 'Birth defects'.
77 J. D. Rainer and F. J. Kallmann, 'Preventive mental health planning', in Rainer, Altshuler, and Kallmann (eds), *Family and Mental Health*, pp. 217–27, here p. 217.
78 Kallmann, *Twin Studies*, pp. 246, 263.
79 See e.g. Kallmann, 'Genetic research', p. 254.
80 K. Z. Altshuler, G. S. Baroff, and J. D. Rainer, 'Operational description of pilot clinic', in Rainer, Altshuler, and Kallmann (eds), *Family and Mental Health*, pp. 155–66, here p. 164–5.
81 Rainer, 'Introduction', p. xiv.
82 Kallmann, 'Genetic aspects', p. 641.
83 See B. R. Hoffman, *Health Care for Some: Rights and Rationing in the United States since 1930* (Chicago, IL: University of Chicago Press, 2013), pp. 41–62, 144–66.

84 See J. M. Loyd, *Health Rights Are Civil Rights: Peace and Justice Activism in Los Angeles, 1963–1978* (Minneapolis, MN: University of Minnesota Press, 2014), pp. 1–18; A. Nelson, *Body and Soul: The Black Panther Party and the Fight Against Medical Discrimination* (Minneapolis, MN: University of Minnesota Press, 2011).
85 Rainer and Kallmann, 'Preventative mental health planning', p. 217.
86 Kallmann, *Twin Studies*, pp. 2, 248.
87 *Ibid.*, p. 96.
88 K. Z. Altshuler, 'The psychiatric preventive programs in a school for the deaf', in Rainer and Altshuler (eds), *Psychiatry and the Deaf*, pp. 11–23, here p. 20.
89 G. C. Kinloch, *The Sociology of Minority Group Relations* (Englewood Cliffs, NJ: Prentice-Hall, 1979), p. 162.
90 See e.g. R. R. Grinker, *Psychiatric Diagnosis, Therapy, and Research on the Psychotic Deaf: Final Report, September 1, 1969* (Washington, DC: U.S. Department of Health, Education, and Welfare, Social Rehabilitation Service, Rehabilitation Services Administration, 1971), p. 8; J. D. Schein, *The Deaf Community: Studies in the Social Psychology of Deafness* (Washington DC: Gallaudet College Press, 1968).
91 For Kallmann's research on homosexuality see e.g. F. J. Kallmann, 'Twin and sibship study of overt male homosexuality', *American Journal of Human Genetics*, 4:2 (1953), 136–46. For his work in the context of research of twins and sexual orientation see. N. H. Boltseridge, 'Identical confusion: the history of twin studies on sexual orientation 1952–1973' (MA thesis, Oregon State University, 2004).

4

PREVENTING TRAGEDY, NEGOTIATING NORMALCY: THE CHANGING MEANING OF USHER SYNDROME, 1960–1980

It was not a geneticist, but a hearing-sighted psychologist, McCay Vernon, who, in the late 1960s, defined Usher syndrome as a distinct genetic form of deaf-blindness – an incurable, hereditary, neuropsychiatric 'chronic incapacitating disease'[1] – and rallied for its eugenic prevention. In doing so, he both perpetuated eugenic and ableist motives, and helped engender an Usher syndrome community that would reject these motives at least partially. The following, then, is not offered as the story of a 'big man' who 'fixed' a disability, but as one of changing and challenged assumptions about what deaf-blind people can and cannot achieve, and what the priorities in dealing with Usher syndrome should be. Inherited in a recessive pattern, Usher syndrome is characterized by congenital hearing loss and progressive vision loss, which usually starts in a person's late childhood or teenage years. The vision loss is due to retinitis pigmentosa, a form of retina degeneration, which results in increasing tunnel vision and eventual legal (though rarely total) blindness. Rare in the general population, it affects circa 3 to 6 per cent of American deaf people.[2]

With such negotiations over what it meant to be deaf and deaf-blind, to have a heritable and progressive condition, the history of Usher syndrome moves at the intersection of patient, disability, and Deaf history, the history of genetics and biomedicine. The 1960s and 1970s were decades of increasingly political and publicly visible Deaf and disability activism. The history of this activism has often been written as inherently opposed to the medical establishment and its pathologizing definitions.[3] Yet it is important to acknowledge that in an era in which the situation of American minorities was very much on people's minds, activism also provided attractive perspectives for medical or rehabilitation professionals. With deafness in particular, a new generation of (mostly young) hearing professionals began siding with Deaf activists who challenged oralism and rallied for the acceptance of sign language, Deaf community, and culture.

Acknowledging that Deaf culture was attractive to professionals also reveals how close together minority activism, ableism, and eugenic thought can be. Usher syndrome is a case in point. McCay Vernon was a life-long, outspoken, and often uncompromising advocate for sign language and Deaf people's rights. During his long career, he received numerous honors and awards, including the Alice Cogswell Award and an Honorary Doctor of Letters from Gallaudet University in 1973 and 1975 respectively, a declaration of merit from the World Federation of the Deaf in 1975 and the Powrie V. Doctor Chair of Deaf Studies Award from Gallaudet in 1979 and 1980. Yet at the same time as he advocated for sign language and Deaf culture, he considered deaf-blindness a most debilitating disability and assessed deaf-blind individuals' agency and abilities according to his own hearing-sighted assumptions. He was by no means alone in this. Deaf-blindness, Vernon recognized later (with perhaps some insight into his own bias), triggered among the (hearing-)sighted intense fears and rejection.[4] With progressing vision loss, deaf-blind people often found themselves at the margins of the Deaf communities in which they had grown up, and grappled with questions of identity and belonging. At the same time, however, contemporary Deaf and disability activism provided them with the tools and rhetoric to reject pathologizing and limiting portrayals and to assert their rights for a self-determined life.

Vernon first encountered individuals with Usher syndrome while he worked as a teacher at the California School for the Deaf in the late 1950s. Over the following years, he would meet more deaf-blind people, first while working on his psychology PhD thesis on deaf children with multiple disabilities, then as a research associate at Chicago's Michael Reese hospital. He was appalled by their living conditions: into the 1960s and 1970s, they were frequently institutionalized in asylums or psychiatric hospitals with little regard to their needs, abilities, and autonomy. Those who lived with their families fared somewhat better, but, with most families never learning tactile communication, were nevertheless severely isolated.

For Vernon, these encounters with deaf-blind people sparked an intense interest – one that, at first, he did not find reciprocated by other professionals, who thought Usher syndrome too rare a condition to deserve much attention. He countered by declaring it a neglected disease, known for a hundred years, yet irresponsibly ignored. This was more rhetoric than reality, but it hit a nerve. It had indeed been known since the late nineteenth century that retinitis pigmentosa was sometimes inherited together with hearing loss; yet it was also often lumped together with other hereditary or non-hereditary forms of deaf-blindness. Only in the 1950s and 1960s, with rapidly expanding knowledge about syndromic deafness, Usher syndrome became visible as a distinct genetic condition. As we have seen in the last chapter, research of syndromic deafness brought with it the realization that a significant part of the deaf population might be affected by undiagnosed metabolic, sensory, or cardiac conditions; a realization that led to calls for closer medical supervision, early identification, and diagnosis.

Launching an ambitious awareness and prevention campaign, Vernon employed these concerns skilfully, tapping into a general sense of urgency, missed chances, and neglect. Usher syndrome, he wrote, was a grave congenital disability that threatened unborn children, and burdened public health with the cost of care for a group of people whose lives were barely worth living. Thus, the best strategy was to invest in eugenic prevention. Vernon's call for screening all deaf children – duly taken up by the 1980s – implied that being deaf meant being at risk. Yet who and what, exactly, was at risk was an ambiguous matter, and opinions shifted over time. Was it the unimpaired future of the unborn child, the family who was affected by the birth of a child with disabilities, the individual whose life and outlook would change drastically with diagnosis, or public health and the public budget impacted by the cost of care?

By the late 1970s, Usher syndrome was no longer an obscure phenomenon, but had become a condition well known among professionals and deaf people. This was not least because of Vernon's campaigning, helped by his growing professional influence – he had become an eminent figure in the psychology of deafness, and, simultaneously, an influential advocate for deaf people's rights. In the 1980s, still, he had (co)authored most publications on Usher syndrome, and was quoted as a major reference in the remainder. The success of his campaigning, however, also brought a greater diversity of stakeholders into the debate, with their own perspectives and agendas. In particular, deaf-blind people themselves became part of the conversation, and challenged the common portrayal of deaf-blindness as hopeless misery. This portrayal still is prevalent today. Both in the popular mind and in professional literature, deaf-blindness is usually seen as the combined effects of deafness and blindness – *Those in Dark Silence*, as a 1930 survey put it.[5] Often based more on hearing-sighted stereotypes than on lived realities, these depictions cast deaf-blind individuals as passive, isolated, and helpless, and tend to negate their ability and autonomy. Deaf-blind advocates, on the other hand, have put forward a portrayal of Usher syndrome that emphasized ability, autonomy, and human variation instead of defect and dependency.

A comprehensive twentieth-century history of deaf-blindness and deaf-blind people is beyond the scope of this chapter, although there is much need for one, beyond a few available (auto)biographies. Looking in this chapter at individuals with Usher syndrome, it is not my intention to universalize their identities and experience as that of all deaf-blind people. Certainly, despite sensory and generational similarities, their experiences and challenges were different than, for example, the children born with chronic rubella syndrome during the 1964–1965 epidemic. And certainly, like in the deaf and disability communities at large, race and class mattered, but were obscured by the fact that attention and resources were granted mostly to white middle-class professionals and advocates. Moreover, as will become clear, even in the period from the 1960s to the 1980s, both who was identified as having Usher syndrome, and the agency granted to and demanded by deaf-blind people, changed significantly. Today, with a growing pro-tactile movement and their twenty-first-century forms of activism and community-building, experiences, identities, and possibilities have changed again.[6]

Taking into account different hearing-sighted, deaf, and deaf-blind perspectives, this chapter follows transformations in what it meant to have Usher syndrome from the 1960s to the 1980s. Unlike previous chapters, which looked at genetic deafness generally, it will focus on a single syndromic form which makes visible larger changes in talking about deafness, disability, and genetics. At stake in discussions about Usher syndrome and those living with it were ideas about genetic risk, prevention, and awareness, and of belonging and identity in the face of changing sensory abilities, professional authority, and patient autonomy. As professionals, deaf, and deaf-blind people debated these issues, the meaning, boundaries, and supposed nature of Usher syndrome changed, as did the prospects of those living with it. By the early 1980s, professionals, too, concentrated mostly on improving living conditions and access to services. In doing so, they replaced the earlier focus on genetic risk and eugenic prevention with an intense interest in the emotional impact of deaf-blindness on the individual and family. Usher syndrome, then, had become a psychological as much as a genetic condition – and geneticists played an important role in this psychologization.

Neglected disease, neglected 'victims': Usher syndrome as a neuropsychiatric condition

Usher syndrome, Vernon kept repeating throughout the 1960s and 1970s, was a tragic condition that had been known and ignored for over a century.[7] This was more a dramatic hyperbole indicting public 'inertia' than a realistic appraisal of past failures. Researchers had, indeed, first noted in the 1850s that hearing loss and retinitis pigmentosa often occurred together, yet Usher syndrome in the modern sense was only defined in the 1960s. Because it is inherited in a recessive manner, and can be traced with relative ease, retinitis pigmentosa had long been a popular research object for ophthalmologists and heredity researchers, and became one of the first model diseases of genetics. In 1914, Scottish ophthalmologist Charles Usher presented a comprehensive study of sixty-nine cases of retinitis pigmentosa, including eleven 'deaf-mutes' and nineteen cases of hearing loss. Like with many eponyms, however, he did not actually define the syndrome ultimately named after him.[8] Rather, it was only the advances in syndromic deafness research in the 1950s and 1960s that made this particular form of deaf-blindness stand out more or less distinctly against similar forms of syndromic deafness. Into the 1970s, still, professionals used the term Usher syndrome inconsistently or not at all, or confused it with other, vaguely similar syndromes.[9]

This relative obscurity was the state of knowledge when McCay Vernon first encountered people with Usher syndrome. Wanting to learn more, he reached out, in 1967, to geneticists, ophthalmologists, and other professionals working with deaf people, asking them to share their research on retinitis pigmentosa. He wrote, for example, to Kenneth Brown, asking for a reprint of his 1966 Clarke School study on genetic deafness. To University of Hawaii geneticist Ian Shine he explained his background and motives: 'Unfortunately, my lack of competence in factors of heredity do not permit me to understand or study the processes of genetic transmission as much as I would like. Instead I have tried to study behavioral and other neuropsychological manifestations of those genetically deafened'.[10] This 'neuropsychological' angle was the focus of Usher syndrome research in the late 1960s and early 1970s.

Many individuals with Usher syndrome, Vernon reported later, had 'spent years of their lives in hospitals for the mentally ill where they were shut away in attics, or in homes where nobody knew how to serve them or to communicate with them'.[11] Psychiatric hospitals and asylums had long been places that warehoused individuals with disabilities not served by special education and rehabilitation, in particular those with multiple or intellectual disabilities. By the 1950s, however, these institutions became the focus of intense criticism that lambasted inhumane living conditions and lack of staff and care. Deinstitutionalization and community services was one answer to this crisis, aiming to rehabilitate patients into society. And it was in this process of psychiatric reform and deinstitutionalization that institutionalized deaf-blind individuals, too, were 'discovered' as a distinct group in need of services.

With psychiatric care for deaf people, the NYSPI mental health project explored in the last chapter had an immense influence. It was duplicated and pushed further elsewhere. One of these locations was Chicago's Michael Reese hospital, where McCay Vernon spent formative years early in his research career. It was here that he encountered more deaf-blind patients, and defined, in 1969, Usher syndrome as an incurable, hereditary, neuropsychiatric 'chronic incapacitating disease'.[12] The Michael Reese project was established in 1965, after a group of psychiatrists and psychologists from Chicago, Vernon included, had travelled to a meeting held by the NYSPI to see the 'world's first and only state mental hospital program for deaf mentally ill patients'. Touring the facilities and talking to project staff, they became '"infected" by the enthusiasm of those concerned with deafness'.[13] These reactions from the Michael Reese group once more make clear how new and exciting the notion of specialized, community-based mental health services for deaf people were to professionals. Impressed by what they saw, the Michael Reese group decided to establish specialized psychosocial services for deaf people in Chicago, too.[14] With two successive grants from the Department of Health, Education, and Welfare Social Rehabilitation Service, covering the period from 1965 to 1969, the project offered professional training and services, such as outpatient and inpatient mental health care or a preschool program for deaf children.[15] Supervised by eminent neuropsychiatrist and psychoanalyst Roy Grinker and led by Vernon, the project team also took part in psychiatric research. Like at the NYSPI, then, research of (syndromic) genetic deafness occurred in a psychiatric institution interested in basic research, psychiatric reform, and community outreach.

Researchers at the NYSPI had gradually come to define deaf people as a sociocultural and linguistic minority. The Chicago group, established ten years later, started with this definition and made it more explicitly political. Vernon, certainly, was a significant influence here. Like Hilde Schlesinger and Edna Levine, two other pioneers in the psychology of deafness, he had entered psychology via deaf education. Born in 1923, he began his career as a teacher, coach, and residence hall counsellor at the Florida, Texas, and Colorado Schools for the Deaf. While working as a teacher, he earned an MS in Education of the Deaf at Gallaudet University in 1954, and an MA in psychology from Florida State University in 1957. He also had private ties to the Deaf community to which his first wife, Edith Goldston Vernon, deaf herself, introduced him. With his background in special education and psychology, he worked as a research associate at the University of Illinois Institute for Research on Exceptional Children while he pursued his PhD research at Claremont Graduate School. His PhD thesis analysed the connection between etiology and intelligence in multiply disabled deaf children.[16] Exploring the intellectual and emotional development of deaf children remained a dominant theme in his career – and marks his ambivalence between advocating for deaf people as a sociolinguistic minority and trying to define deaf pathologies.

Borrowing from the radicalizing language of civil rights and minority movements, the Michael Reese group criticized majority society for oppressing the language and culture of deaf people. 'The average deaf youth', Grinker wrote for example, was part of 'a minority group that is more often the butt of crude humor than of understanding'. He was 'generally forced to communicate through a "foreign" language and modality, his natural language (the language of signs) being forbidden'.[17] Grinker's condemnation echoed the analysis presented by psychologist Hilde Schlesinger at a 1968 NYSPI meeting, which he had attended. There she had theorized about the estrangement that deaf children experienced when 'one of their native tongues' – sign language – 'is not quite so good, not quite as acceptable, as the spoken language'.[18]

Vernon similarly compared the situation of deaf people with that of other ethnic minorities. Mirroring contemporary beliefs about model minorities and ethnic identity, he concluded that those groups who succeeded in American society – Catholics, Jews, Mormons, and 'Orientals' – had developed strategies to maintain their identity and autonomy. Others – 'Puerto Ricans, Negroes and American Indians' – who remained disadvantaged, were marked by their 'second class citizenship', and were told that their culture and language were undesirable.[19] The 'effort to deprive and make deaf persons ashamed of manual communication and other aspects of themselves as deaf people', he wrote, 'have analogues in the hair straightening, skin bleaching and other examples of minority group attempts to deny their identities and become something they are not'. In the politically charged atmosphere of the late 1960s, thus evoking the oppression of African and Native Americans was a powerful tool to mark oralist education as an undemocratic aberration.[20]

At the same time – and often contradicting their own definition of deaf people as a sociocultural group – Vernon and the Michael Reese group delineated the supposed psychopathological effects of deafness. Like the NYSPI researchers, they were interested in defining how deaf and hearing people's emotional and intellectual development differed, and in whether these differences resulted in particular psychiatric disturbances. Yet where the NYSPI had defined deafness as a 'stress-producing' psychosocial condition, they located deaf people's supposed difference in their neurological make-up, their brains.

Vernon in particular pushed this notion in his influential research on intelligence and educational achievement. 'Brain damage', he wrote in 1971, 'plays a major role in a significant number of the behavior disorders in deaf persons'. There was, he claimed, a critical overlap between the most common causes of deafness and of brain damage: maternal rubella, meningitis, prematurity, heredity, and serological complications. Consequently the 'behavior noted as characteristic for deaf persons may not be caused by deafness at all' but rather by an 'interaction between central nervous system damage and deafness'.[21] Where these neurological lesions supposedly occurred, and how they would actually affect neurological function, remained purely speculative. Yet neurology offered an attractive model for locating – in the supposed concreteness of brain matter – the cause for differences in deaf people's educational achievements or social adaptation. For Vernon, Usher syndrome, too, was one such example of sensory and neuropsychiatric impairment.

Vernon's attempt to diagnose deaf people with some undefined brain damage has often – and rightly so – been considered offensive. Harlan Lane, for example, himself a psychologist and eminent advocate for Deaf culture, criticized this 'inferred brain lesions' as an example for the medicalization of deafness.[22] This is certainly true. Yet Vernon's insistence on neurological damage as the *real* cause for deaf difference is also part of a longer tradition in the history of deafness, disability, and eugenics. Faced with accusations of inferior otherness, social deviance, or educational underachievement, minorities have often reacted by emphasizing their middle-class respectability, normalcy, and ability, in turn excluding those who did not fit these criteria. The deaf community was no exception, as Susan Burch and Octavian Robinson have pointed out.[23]

In hindsight, it is difficult to reconcile Vernon's advocacy for Deaf culture and sign language with his search for deaf neuropathology and eugenic solutions for Usher syndrome. He and his contemporaries, however, did not operate with the binary opposition of a medical-pathological and a socio-cultural model of deafness or disability that has become prevalent in early twenty-first century disability history and activism. Rather, they moved and meandered between these poles, sometimes thinking of it as a matter of positivist science and medicine, sometimes as one of social bias and discrimination, justice and civil rights. From which framework they drew depended on, in part, the valence it held within a particular professional or social context, and which audience was addressed. Significantly, by the 1960s, deaf people had become one of these audiences, at least to some professionals; a community one spoke to – in their own language – not only about.

This was not (yet) true for deaf-blind people. They were an unknown entity, a group whose condition was unimaginable to hearing-sighted professionals. Looking at deaf-blindness from their own perspectives, these professionals tended to reproduce ableist hierarchies and assumptions prevalent both within the hearing and deaf worlds. Certainly, this perception was shaped by the deaf-blind asylum patients that came to the attention of professionals in the 1960s. Most of them had been neglected and isolated for years, even decades. Frequently (and unsurprisingly, given this neglect), they also showed intellectual delay and behavioural or mental health issues. For researchers, this posed a puzzling problem. They discussed intensely whether these psychiatric and intellectual problems were an innate part of deaf-blindness or caused by it.[24] Unlike some of his colleagues, who saw no causal relation, Vernon defined Usher syndrome as a neuropsychiatric condition. He framed this definition with his larger theory of brain lesions causing behavioural difference among deaf people: in Usher syndrome, he believed, both vision and hearing loss and the psychiatric traits were caused by a – speculative and yet to be discovered – 'central nervous system damage'.[25] This was a definition upon which he built his prevention plan, and which he would uphold until encounters with deaf-blind people outside institutional walls brought about a less deterministic notion of sensory difference and psychosocial response.

Hopeless fates and bright individuals: the changing face of deaf-blindness

In 1969, Vernon published an extensive action plan to raise awareness for Usher syndrome and to eventually eradicate it. As he explained in various articles and in correspondence with individuals, organizations, and federal agencies, spreading awareness was the first step for further measures, in particular the screening of all congenitally deaf children – the high-risk group for undiagnosed Usher syndrome. Among them, he claimed, the syndrome was the leading cause of deaf-blindness. Conveniently, this risk population was 'small, identified, centralized and available' in schools for the deaf. Setting up a programme of detection and genetic counselling for them and their family members in order 'to avert further spread of the disease' thus was both 'feasible and potentially effective'.[26]

In his crusade for the eradication of Usher syndrome, Vernon often skilfully used the dehumanizing language of economic cost, suffering, and misery that has long dominated public and scientific conversations about disability. The cost of prevention, he argued, 'would be infinitesimal compared to the cost of educating, training, or even merely providing custodial care for a deaf-blind person'. The cost of educating one deaf-blind child – $182,000 in 1976 – would be 'enough to pay for several years of nation-wide screening'. These were harsh words from a former teacher for the deaf. Genetic screening and counselling, he acknowledged, may 'pose many ethical and philosophical problems', yet when 'the drawbacks of counseling are weighted against the awesome nature of deaf-blindness it is apparent that they are the lesser evil'.[27] Research, too, could be cast in the depersonalized language of economic savings versus current misspending and failed investment in public health. In this line of arguing, finding a cure or an in utero test would be 'cost-effective in that the expenditures would not approach the cost of maintaining even minimal services for deaf-blind people'.[28]

Often harshly uncompromising and impatient about seeing his prevention plan implemented, Vernon found to his frustration that other deafness professionals considered Usher syndrome just one problem among many that demanded their attention. With deaf-blindness in particular, it was the 1964–1965 rubella epidemic that captured public attention, not unlike the last polio epidemic a decade earlier. The US alone registered 12.5 million cases. Usually mild in children and adults, rubella (or German measles), a viral infection, poses a serious threat to the unborn. It can cause Congenital Rubella Syndrome (CRS), which most commonly includes a distinctive combination of cataracts, hearing loss, and congenital heart disease.[29] During the 1964–1965 epidemic, 11,000 pregnant women who had contracted rubella either miscarried or aborted once they learned of the damaging effects. Between 20,000 and 30,000 babies were born with CRS, among them 2,500 to 4,400 with deaf-blindness.[30]

The dilemma of pregnant women who contracted rubella and the fate of the children born with CRS grabbed public attention. Leslie Reagan has argued that the rubella epidemic acted as a catalyst for debates over abortion, public health, and disability. Before the legalization of abortion, access for rubella-infected pregnant women varied widely, depending on location, race, and social position. Often, women were denied abortions, or had to fight their case until very late in their pregnancy, an experience that galvanized many of them into lobbying for legalization. At the same time, parents of children with CRS played an important role in advocating for better services, education, and social acceptance.[31] Here, there was significant progress. At schools for the deaf, educators tried to anticipate the needs of the rubella cohort, which was about three to five times the number of the average deaf-blind school population. In 1967, the Vocational Rehabilitation Act Amendment acknowledged, for the first time, deaf-blind people's suitability for vocational rehabilitation. In 1976, the Helen Keller National Center (HKC) for Deaf-Blind Youths and Adults opened its doors in Sands Points, New York. It offered rehabilitation and training services and facilities. Ten regional Centers for Deaf-Blind Children supported the national centre.[32]

There are some striking similarities in the perception of CRS and Usher syndrome: both were portrayed as a 'human burden'[33] or an 'unnecessary tragedy';[34] the former to be prevented through vaccination, the latter via genetic awareness and counselling. With both, professionals contrasted the low cost of prevention with the familial, financial, and social resources for the education and rehabilitation of the 'damaged' child.[35] Yet there were also important differences. 'The new "handicapped" child born of German measles', Reagan writes, 'were [sic] pitied not only because they had disabilities but also because their expected prosperous future had been interrupted'.[36] Children with Usher syndrome, on the other hand, were seen as disabled from conception, although vision loss only manifested itself later in life.

The meaning of prevention also differed. With the discovery of the rubella virus in 1962 and consequent development of a vaccine, maternal rubella became an easily preventable condition. Large-scale vaccination campaigns followed. By 1978 almost all states in the US had made rubella vaccination mandatory for school children. By 1984, rubella was considered contained.[37] Usher syndrome, on the other hand, remains an incurable condition. Then, as now, biochemical research raised hopes for future treatments. In the 1960s, the model condition for these hopes was Phenylketonuria (PKU). The realization that a diet low in phenylalanine could prevent and even reverse the severe developmental delay of untreated PKU was a major breakthrough, and led to widespread new-born screening.[38] The discovery that Refsum disease – another, rarer form of hereditary retinitis pigmentosa and hearing loss with neurological symptoms – could, similarly, be treated with dietary restrictions raised expectations for a similar intervention with Usher syndrome. Yet, as with most genetic conditions, such scientific successes remained elusive. When it came to Usher syndrome, prevention meant finding affected individuals and non-affected recessive carriers in order to 'treat' them with genetic counselling and, potentially, 'therapeutic' abortion.

Although Vernon's main audience was other professionals, he also published in venues that primarily addressed deaf or blind lay people.[39] This had unexpected consequences. Soon, he began receiving letters from individuals, who, after reading one of these pieces, realized that they or a family member had Usher syndrome. For some, it was only after reading one of these articles that they learned the name or full extent of their condition. For these correspondents, Vernon came to act as a confidant who provided comfort, information, and referrals to experts and services. In 1974, for example, a mother from Florida complained that even though her son had been diagnosed with Usher syndrome, the diagnosing physician had failed to give them any relevant information. Vernon replied empathetically. 'You face some difficult times in helping your son get the most he can from life'. He offered the mother 'any help I can'.[40] For other correspondents, realizing the hereditary nature of their condition raised questions about marriage and childbearing. A concerned mother wrote to Vernon in 1974, asking for more information on behalf of her deaf son and deaf-blind daughter in law. He directed her to John D. Rainer who now headed the NYSPI Department of Medical Genetics.[41]

These points of contact with the hopes, feelings, and expectation of his correspondents changed Vernon's portrayal of Usher syndrome. Prevention remained a primary concern, yet the focus shifted from the abstract language of eugenics, public health, and economic savings to the psychosocial impact on the individual and family. Many of his correspondents, he realized, 'were bright, successful individuals, who, in some cases, were hard of hearing and partially sighted rather than severely deaf-blind'. Their existence, he concluded, pointed to a bias in research. Earlier studies, including his own, had focused on deaf-blind individuals who lived in institutions, and on whom decades of neglect had left their mark. Now it became apparent that there was a group of people with Usher syndrome in whom vision loss was not (yet) severe, who were often accomplished professionals, and who had adapted to their situation, living fulfilling 'normal' lives.[42]

Families at risk? From eugenic prevention to psychosocial genetic counselling

By the late 1970s, awareness of Usher syndrome had grown significantly, thanks to a variety of forces, including the expanding network around Vernon's awareness campaign, and the growing attention to the needs of deaf children with additional disabilities. Schools for the deaf had improved services for deaf-blind children and began implementing screening programmes for vision problems. Deaf children thus became a group targeted for mass screening that did not aim at the general population, but at a specific group with a particularly high prevalence of a certain condition, such as Tay Sachs disease among Ashkenazi Jewish populations, or sickle cell disease among African Americans.[43] By 1981, twenty-one of fifty-nine residential schools had such screening programmes. Half of them also offered support services, personal, vocational, and genetic counselling, or curricular modifications.[44]

Throughout the 1970s and early 1980s, the question of how to best serve deaf-blind people brought together professionals from various fields with deaf-blind individuals and family members. At various meetings, workshops, and conferences, they discussed screening, diagnosis, and genetic counselling; how to improve services, education, and rehabilitation; and the personal, social, and emotional implications of living with deaf-blindness. What happened to deaf individuals who learned that they would lose their vision, how did their families react? How could professionals help them cope, what services should be offered? Increasingly, it was these psychosocial dimensions of Usher syndrome that claimed professional attention; a development that would have a significant impact on genetic counselling, too. Usher syndrome came to be seen as a threat to the emotional equilibrium of the individual and their family. In order to prevent lasting emotional damage, professionals claimed, they required continuous psychological supervision and support.

The moment of diagnosis was given particular attention. It was a potentially damaging moment of transformation from healthy to disabled. (It is noteworthy how here being deaf became the normal, healthy state.) As individuals with Usher syndrome came under intense scrutiny, even 'normal' behaviour became a potential sign of emotional disturbance. Ed Hammer, director of the South Central Regional Center for Services to Deaf-Blind Children, for example, emphasized that emotional distress was not only normal, it was a necessary stage in the process of coping. He advised in 1978 that '[g]reater concern needs to be given to the person who does not experience "mini-psychosis"' when finding out about their vision loss. This, he cautioned, 'may be the person who is out of touch with reality'.[45] Similarly, Vernon, together with geneticist Joann Boughman, and Linda Annala, herself living with Usher syndrome, wrote in 1982: 'The entire psychodynamic process of coping with the diagnosis is life-long, extremely difficult, and changes as the persons grows older and the visual loss progresses'.[46]

The moment of diagnosis received even more attention when, with new vision screening programmes in schools for the deaf, the age of diagnosis decreased. Where before, people receiving a diagnosis had been young or middle-aged adults, who had often already experienced significant vision loss, it was now children and teenagers in whom it was not yet profound. Lowering the age of diagnosis was seen as a success, but it also brought new ethical questions and anxieties. Learning about the diagnosis was upsetting even to adults but much more troubling with children and teenagers. They were considered a particularly vulnerable group. Parents and professionals feared that learning about their impending vision loss might cause emotional damage. Moreover, parents were under emotional pressure themselves. It was usually parents who first learned about the diagnosis, and were put in the difficult position of passing it on to their children. But when was a child or a teenager old enough to know that they would lose their vision? During the late 1970s and early 1980s, parents and professionals debated emotionally the when and how of telling children and teenagers about Usher syndrome. They weighed prevention against emotional stability; timely adaptation against the impact of learning about vision loss; plans and hopes in the present against future impairment.[47]

Communicating the diagnosis to parents standing in for their children reinforced the character of Usher syndrome as an intergenerational condition, something that affected – and potentially harmed – the relationship between parents, the affected child, and potentially their siblings. From such a psychosocial angle, it posed a range of emotional challenges for the affected person and their family. It was, professionals emphasized, an interconnected condition that required the entire family to accept loss and limitations, and to learn about new options and ways of doing things. Observing affected families, Carolyn Torrie, a counsellor from the University of Texas South Central Regional Center for Deaf-Blind Children, pointed out their particularly difficult situation. When their child was born, they had to come to terms with their deafness; a confusing and often difficult adaption. Nevertheless, they had eventually found some kind of emotional equilibrium. Now, the realization that their son or daughter would also lose their vision rekindled 'old feelings of grief, pain and anger'. In this situation, counsellors could encourage new coping mechanisms and 'enable them to learn that all is not hopeless for their children, that their lives do not have to develop into emptiness'. For deaf-blind children and adolescents, she recommended group counselling programmes where they could 'share their anxieties, despair, anger and concerns' and 'learn to take strength from the mutuality of their concerns for each other'.[48]

There was an additional, genetic dimension to these concerns about coping and acceptance. If the affected person and their family failed at this task, some professionals feared, they not only endangered their own future, but also that of the unborn next generation. Emotional coping thus became a precondition for rational family planning. Unless the affected teenager and his or her parents 'can handle these stages of adjustment', Torrie wrote for example, 'they will not take on the burden of accepting Usher's syndrome as an inherited disorder, with the implication of this in questions such as producing more victims'.[49] Such language portrayed the syndrome as an unrelenting aggressor, yet also suggested that one could and should prepare against it.

Torrie's emphasis on the psychological readiness for genetic knowledge was common in contemporary genetics. With the shift towards non-directed counselling, geneticists observed and tried to make sense of client's reactions to genetic information, and reimagined counselling as an emotional process, only at the end of which there could be a truly rational and informed decision. They pointed to the psycho-emotional benefits of genetic knowledge as a means to be ready for life's challenges. This emphasis on psycho-emotional dimensions was an ambivalent development. It did not necessarily negate eugenic beliefs about disability or restrictive definitions of the 'normal family'. Rather, it shows a shift in expectations about what genetics could achieve, and how different professions imagined these goals differently. For Vernon, the psychologist, genetic counselling was primarily a eugenic tool to eradicate Usher syndrome. This goal was more important than individual hopes for children or marriage. Geneticists, on the other hand, had been moving away from this absolute stance. Disease prevention and public health remained important goals in genetics, yet by mid-century, geneticists had realized that preventing a trait or gene at the individual level really would not do much to lower its frequency in the total population. This was particularly true for recessive genes, where many unaffected carriers, with just one affected gene, would never know, unless they had children with another carrier. Instead, they focused on the situation of the individual, couple, or family.

Walter Nance's position is a good example. A leading expert on genetic deafness, he became involved in the Usher syndrome community in the 1970s. Speaking at a 1973 Gallaudet symposium on Usher syndrome, he explained that the psychotherapeutic benefits of counselling were superior to its medical or eugenic effects. Unlike Vernon, who disapproved of marriages of individuals with Usher syndrome, Nance encouraged them to be 'optimistic', as their chances for unaffected children were much better than generally assumed. (Since it is a recessive trait, a child will only have Usher syndrome if both parents are affected.) Genetics, he believed, echoing a common theme in genetic counselling, could dispel such fears created by misinformation, social bias, and ignorance. He assured patients and their families that 'the load of abnormal recessive genes is a burden that all society bears'. Given this ubiquity, 'the social stigma that was formerly attached to genetic diseases of all types can be seen to be a reflection of ignorance'.[50] Much more than merely a science of prevention, genetics was to be a gateway science, opening a path for a more aware – and thus more self-determined – (family) life.

Other professionals were caught between the desire to acknowledge patient autonomy and non-directiveness, and their own ideas about the 'right outcome'. Preventing Usher syndrome, explained University of Texas obstetrician-gynaecologist M. J. E. Harrod in 1977, 'is one important goal of counselling, but more important by far are the goals of understanding and responsible decision making that counseling can promote'. Harrod, too, emphasized the need for psychological readiness, without which those affected would be unable to understand the implications of the diagnosis. Giving too much information too soon, on the other hand, would likely result in 'a counseling failure' – an uninformed reproductive decision.[51] Describing this situation, Harrod found himself in a basic dilemma of non-directive counselling: how to deal with decisions that deviated from one's own beliefs and goals. Although he believed that there were 'no "wrong" decisions ... as long as they are truly informed decisions', he maintained that 'parenthood is out of the question for that [deaf-blind] individual, regardless of his or her own feelings about the issue'. Deaf-blind people, in other words, did not make for good, responsible parents. Their autonomy was only granted within the limits of professionally approved reproductive decisions.[52]

Looking at the psycho-emotional state of individuals with Usher syndrome, then, simultaneously facilitated more client-centred narratives, and professional claims that they knew best how to deal with difficult emotional situations. Risk remained a central concept, yet by the mid-1970s, the understanding of risk had moved from the body to the psyche, and from the single, isolated, or institutionalized person to an individual within a family, often a child or teenager. What before the diagnosis had been a 'normal' family, now was one that needed constant professional and self-surveillance for signs of emotional disturbance, deviance, and maldevelopment. Families with an affected person shared an at-risk status, which was founded as much on the emotional impact of deaf-blindness as on the actual genetic connection between family members. Notably, this continuum of psychological risk did not necessarily map upon the progress of vision loss, or, indeed, genetic risk. Finally, this psychologized mode of thinking about risk and life with Usher syndrome also influenced the emerging identities and narratives of affected individuals, although they would give it a more self-determined spin.

Coming 'to grips with having Usher's': self-discovery and self-realization

Into the second half of the twentieth century, hearing-sighted professionals had spoken about, but not with deaf people. This was even truer for deaf-blind people, to whom professionals and the general public hardly ever granted full human potential and agency. Yet by the 1970s and 1980s, conferences, workshops, and correspondence brought together hearing-sighted, deaf, and deaf-blind professionals, patients, and advocates. Here, deaf-blind individuals began shaping the conversation about Usher syndrome with their demands for self-determination and independence, and their emphasis on ability instead of defect. Where professionals portrayed low achievement, isolation, and restrictions as the natural side-effects of deaf-blindness, deaf-blind people themselves emphasized that it was mostly bias and discrimination that limited their participation in social and professional life.

In this first generation of Usher syndrome advocates two people stand out: Arthur Roehrig and Linda Annala (1948–2007). Until her death in 2007, Annala was active in the Louisiana deaf-blind community, where Usher syndrome is particularly prevalent in the Cajun population.[53] Roehrig, too, has been a public advocate for deaf-blind people. He worked as a counsellor and coordinator for deaf-blind people at the Gallaudet Public Service Program and later served as the long-time president of the American Association of the Deaf-Blind (AADB). Their background and path to diagnosis was similar and typical. Both had graduated from schools for the deaf and started careers as teachers. Despite early signs of decreasing vision, both were only diagnosed as adults. They also identified as part of the Deaf community, an identity that was questioned with their vision loss.

Looking back at the time before their diagnosis, both Annala and Roehrig pointed to the anxiety and confusion caused by their gradual and unexplained vision loss. The diagnosis initiated a long process of coping with their identity, of finding a new sense of belonging to a larger community of deaf-blind people. At a 1976 Helen Keller Center workshop, Annala for example shared how she 'came to grips with having Usher's'. Looking back, she could not remember specifically when her vision began to deteriorate, although as a teenager she found it 'frustrating and difficult' to be the only one among her friends who could not follow signed conversations in dimly lit places. Some years later, her friends pointed out that she might have tunnel vision, a suspicion she 'promptly denied ... because I could see sideways'. She had her eyes checked nevertheless, yet the ophthalmologists dismissed her as having 'nerves'. In hindsight, she identified several other such missed moments, where her own desire to ignore her vision problems combined with professional ignorance or dismissal.[54]

With a BA from Gallaudet and a Master's in deaf education from Western Maryland College – one of the few colleges which at the time admitted deaf graduates – she began working as a teacher at the Illinois School for the Deaf in Jacksonville. Her friends remained concerned about her vision. In 1973, after two of them had read an article on Usher syndrome in *Gallaudet Today*, the school's alumni newsletter, they recognized the symptoms in Annala, and asked her to see an eye specialist. First, however, she 'tried a simple experiment'. Wriggling her fingers at the side of her head, she was surprised to find that she could not see her hand from some angles. In this moment of self-diagnosis, she 'realized that this was the "tunnel vision" my friends were trying to tell me about'.[55]

Her self-diagnosis, however, was not confirmed by the ophthalmologist she consulted. His failure to check her field of vision provided a temporary reprieve – until one month later she had a car accident because of her tunnel vision. She dismissed this event, yet in early 1974, when she went through a spiritual conversion, she 'asked the Lord to either heal my vision or give me the name of the abnormality and to guide me'. She received an answer that was as clear as it was unwanted: another car accident.[56] Shortly after, she came across an article on Usher syndrome in the *Deaf American*, the official NAD publication. Facing a written description of her symptoms finally provided enough points of identification. After talking to her friends, she decided to give up driving and 'to face the future with this eye condition known as "Usher's Syndrome"'. Self-diagnosis and acceptance thus preceded the official medical diagnosis, which she received a bit later from a Jacksonville eye specialist.[57]

Roehrig's path to diagnosis was very similar, although his narrative drew more explicitly from the language of psychology and counselling. In 1973, he described the 'three levels of awareness of deteriorating vision in the victim of Usher's syndrome', from the unconscious to the semi-conscious and finally to diagnosis and acceptance. Like Annala, he had noticed early on that his night vision was worse than that of other students at the St John's School for the Deaf in Milwaukee. For a long time, this caused no problems. By 1971, however, in his second year as a teacher at the Maryland School for the Deaf, his vision had deteriorated to the point where he had trouble following his students' conversations. He had entered a state of being 'semi-consciously aware of my visual impairment'. He became 'depressed and worried', and began seeking professional diagnosis and support.[58]

Talking to a social worker about adjustments to his vision loss, he 'became consciously and hopelessly aware of what would happen to my eyes in the next few years – I mean blindness'. He was 'naturally depressed and cried all night because I knew I would be blind some day'. In hindsight, however, he believed that this realization was 'not as traumatic as some people might think'.[59] Where the conventional narrative saw diagnosis as a tragic and hopeless endpoint, he considered it a stage to be overcome with human resilience. Having Usher syndrome, he realized, 'was neither my fault nor my parents'. It was something he was born with, and eventually nothing more or less than the 'individual differences among all people'.[60] With such universal themes as self-realization and fulfilment, Roehrig appealed to a larger audience, no matter their sensory status. Casting deaf-blindness as an individual variation depathologized it, and turned it into one of life's various challenges on the path towards individual development and growth.

When Roehrig and Annala cast their life with Usher syndrome as a journey towards self-help, self-finding, and self-acceptance, they appealed to themes prevalent in 1970s American culture. In many ways, Roehrig's portrayal of Usher syndrome also was typical for new ways of talking about disability or chronic conditions in the second half of the twentieth century. In the first decades of the century, both professional literature and self-portrayals had focused on 'overcoming' for the sake of good citizenship and economic independence. Now the emphasis was increasingly on the effect of disability on selfhood, identity, and social relations. This was part of a more general interest in self-help, self-finding, and self-acceptance that also became an essential part of biomedicine.[61] Patient movements, Margaret Lock and Vinh-Kim Nguyen have argued, embraced public and private self-examination as a form of self-help and empowerment, creating new identities around a shared condition. Such practices provide a specific form of condition management based on the belief that sharing one's inner self with others is cathartic.[62] Early theorists of disability and identity, such as Irving Zola or Erving Goffman, also contributed to this idea, exploring the mechanism of bias, exclusion, and stigmatization.[63]

Genetics, too, could be employed for portraying life with Usher syndrome as a larger journey towards self-knowledge and self-acceptance. Its attractiveness as a narrative framework for deaf or deaf-blind people makes visible the ironies of genetic education. Like other professionals before him, Vernon had tried to instil in deaf people a eugenic responsibility towards prevention, potentially at the cost of having a family or children of one's own. As an advocate of (an ableist) Deaf culture, he limited these appeals to Usher syndrome. By the 1970s, however, other models of genetic knowledge had become available, not least promoted by geneticists like Nance, for whom the primary goal was not prevention but the emotional benefits of genetic awareness.

In 1975, for example, Nance had collaborated with the Gallaudet Public Service division, publishing a short booklet on heredity and deafness that explicitly addressed a deaf audience 'to help you understand your heredity'. It presented basic information about genetic concepts such as traits and genes, patterns of inheritance and likely scenarios for genetic deafness. Nance, who believed that genetic counselling should be sensitive to Deaf culture, presented heredity as the source of human uniqueness and singularity. He also promoted genetic knowledge as an important means of self-knowledge, of gaining 'a deeper understanding of ourselves'. 'Knowing how traits – any traits – are inherited', he believed, 'is a step forward in understanding ourselves'.[64] The booklet noted that 'each of us carries between four to ten genes that could cause genetic problems'. The ubiquity of mutations in the general population had been a staple theme in genetics since about the 1940s. In genetic counselling, it often served as a soothing message, reassuring parents that their own or their child's condition was not their fault. As Nance put it, 'each of us shares the burden for potential genetic illnesses in the world'. Some genetic variations were harmless, others could cause medical, financial, or social complications. He noted that '[e]motional adjustments to the condition must be made by the individual and his family if he is to live an independent life'. Yet, he emphasized, there was 'nothing wrong with inheriting a genetic condition', no need to 'feel ashamed'. Rather than stumbling unprepared into such a situation, it was useful to acquire a general awareness of the workings of heredity. The important thing was to 'be honest and realistic in coping with the problems a genetic condition may cause'.[65]

Individuals with Usher syndrome picked up on these themes and incorporated them in a more positive portrayal of their condition. 'Every human being', Roehrig wrote for example in 1976, 'has 2 to 7 defective genes'.[66] To him, Nance's portrayal of genetics as a matter of personal adaption and awareness, of finding one's place on a spectrum of human variation, was more appealing than Vernon's urgent call for prevention and restriction. He seized genetic knowledge as a means for normalizing and humanizing his condition. Defective genes were a communality shared with all of humankind, and their expression was merely a matter of chance. It did not devalue the affected person.

'[C]hampion[ing] the cause for others': advocacy and contested identities

For both Annala and Roehrig, diagnosis brought the realization that they were part of a larger group of people with Usher syndrome. In a way, this sense of community was a consequence of expanding screening and diagnosis, of more readily available information. In this development towards community formation, Usher syndrome was no exception. Historians have described how, from the late 1960s on, 'genetic communities' formed around a certain condition, made up of affected individuals, family members, and professionals, rallying for various goals, including search for a treatment, better services, or public awareness.[67] As individuals with Usher syndrome found each other, they became an imagined and increasingly face-to-face community. Here, Annala and Roehrig emerged as spokespersons. For them, acting as advocates provided a sense of purpose. Right after diagnosis, Annala recalled, her future had 'looked dark and dismal'. She decided that it 'would be brighter, if I would champion the cause and improve conditions of people like myself who were deaf and gradually losing their sight'. In doing so, she hoped to 'help make the future more promising for the young people who are now in high school, vocational training programs or in colleges'.[68] This was a pressing concern to Roehrig, too. Attitudes towards deaf-blindness, he stated in 1976 with some resignation, were 'generally very negative and difficult to change'. The 'lack of interest and awareness on the needs of deaf-blind people by the general population', he explained, 'exacerbates the problem of social and personal interaction'.[69]

Finding a community of their own was particularly important to individuals with Usher syndrome who, upon diagnosis, often found themselves between communities and identities. Born with congenital hearing loss, many had attended schools for the deaf, and after graduation took part in Deaf community life. When they began losing their vision and eventually received the diagnosis, they feared exclusion from a highly visual culture and from a community that considered blindness one of the worst disabilities imaginable. This sense of exclusion and not-quite-belonging to neither the deaf nor to the blind community figures prominently in personal narratives. Annala, for example, felt restricted by negative attitudes, in particular 'the aversion on the part of others, particularly deaf people who use sign language, to communicate with the deaf-blind person'.[70]

At the same time, her experience as a member of the Deaf community enabled her to develop a deaf-blind identity and community that sought the connection to Deaf culture. Tactile sign language, for example, allowed continuing communication with deaf friends, family, and co-workers. Annala saw herself as a mediator between the larger Deaf community, to which she had belonged all of her life, and the newer, smaller deaf-blind community. 'As a person who has this disease and as a teacher for the deaf', she explained, 'I want to continue to champion the cause, breaking down the barriers of ignorance and fear on the part of the deaf population'.[71]

Deaf-blind people certainly faced bias and prejudice within the deaf community. At the same time, deaf community leaders were also sensitized to their situation by their own experiences of exclusion and dismissal. Being deaf himself, Albert Pimentel commented in 1976 that he was aware of the limits society placed on deaf-blind people. Pimentel, director of Gallaudet's public service programmes, pointed to deaf education and rehabilitation, which for a long time had been dominated by hearing professionals. Only 'as some of our well-meaning friends retired or finally developed more awareness of currents trends', had deaf people themselves gained more of a chance to influence education and rehabilitation services. In this situation, they had found inspiration and orientation in the activism of other minorities. As 'the Civil Rights Movement for other minorities emboldened some of us to explore the "can't do" areas', he recounted, 'the disability of deafness suddenly became a more manageable handicap for many deaf people'.[72] Now deaf-blind people were in a similar position of lingering paternalism. It was wrong, Pimentel believed, to exclude them from any educational or professional opportunity. Whereas many hearing-sighted professionals focused on exploring deficits, he instead emphasized ability and self-determination. 'With our limited knowledge', he observed, 'it's better at this point to let those with ambition who live with Usher's Syndrome point the way'.[73]

Living with Usher syndrome meant negotiating the borders of disability and difference. This was a matter of individual soul-searching, and of refiguring one's place among family, friends, and in society at large. Like many people who had grown up deaf, Roehrig did not consider deafness a disability. 'Congenital deafness', he generalized about Usher syndrome, 'is accepted easily because the sense of hearing is never experienced'. The prospect of blindness, on the other hand, could be 'traumatic' at first. Yet it, too, was 'usually accepted, although more slowly'.[74] It helped to recall that deaf-blindness was not unique. '[E]very human being can, at any time, become doubly or multiply handicapped'. From this perspective, full hearing and sight was only a temporary state; its disruption a challenge that could be dealt with like other life events. Emphasizing the essential humanity of deaf-blind people, Roehrig believed that a deaf-blind person could 'function as a normal person in most ways despite his double handicap', and had 'every right to live as much of a normal life as possible'.[75] To him, this meant the right to partake in the normal life of the average American, to have a job, friends, and family.

Living with Usher syndrome, Roehrig believed, was manageable and worthwhile if one was willing to adapt, had good support systems, and found a place in society. Being able to lead a self-determined life and finding respect were key issues. That these were also experiences routinely denied to deaf-blind people is apparent in Roehrig's appeal that 'every person with Usher's syndrome wants to be respected primarily as a human being and to be treated like others'.[76] Self-determination, respect, self-help, and independent living, of course, were central demands of disability activism and the self-help movement. It was a practical demand of the students with physical disabilities who during the late 1960s enrolled in colleges against considerable pushback from educators and administrators.[77] Early disability theorists, like Irving K. Zola, also advocated for self-help, and criticized the fact that rehabilitation goals often were shaped more by social expectations than tailored to individual needs and preferences. Self-determination, Zola argued, was a condition for self-respect and a positive self-image.[78]

Bias and prejudice also massively affected employment chances. Roehrig emphasized that the issue was not deaf-blind people's lack of ability, but discrimination and inflexibility on the side of employers and society at large. The main problem was 'that jobs and buildings have been purposefully or inadvertently planned for people who can see, hear, and are highly mobile'. With thirty-six million people with disabilities in the US, however, such presumptions were not acceptable. Identifying with 'people who cannot see, hear, and/or walk', he allied his cause more broadly with that of disability rights activism.[79] Roehrig made his call at a time in the 1970s when disability activism radicalized and drew public attention with acts of civil disobedience. Student and campus activism played an important role, and certainly provided inspiration for Roehrig as well. Once they left college, young disabled professionals brought their experience with battling college administration to a larger political arena, achieving some noteworthy successes.[80]

Historians and activists have sometimes argued that, for the most part, the disability and Deaf movements and communities have mostly gone separate ways. Katherine Jankowski, for example, argues that deaf people have a shared language and culture, and thus are more like an oppressed sociolinguistic group than part of the disability community. The latter, she writes, consists of 'hearing people who have more in common with the general populace than they do with Deaf people'.[81] Certainly, this often captures the self-perception of deaf people or those with disabilities. Yet focusing on such binaries obscures the lived realities of many people with intersecting or conflicting identities.[82]

Usher syndrome is a case in point. Not only did affected individuals go from being deaf to being deaf-blind, and thus to someone who even in their own community was considered gravely disabled. In addition, with their diagnosis and ensuing need for check-ups and assessment, they also found themselves in the role of the patient, in a time in which this role was changing, when traditional medical authority and paternalism became challenged – yet when it was also still very much alive. Individuals with Usher syndrome thus found themselves with three identities – deaf, disabled, and patient – that were contested from within these communities, and by the professionals with which they interacted. As they negotiated difference and ability, these identities intertwined, forming a new sense of belonging.

Their interactions with physicians, geneticists, counsellors, or psychologists offer an example for the ambivalent, complicated, but not necessarily antagonistic relationship between professionals and deaf, disability, and patient movements. Historians have often focused on the opposition between these movements and established science and medicine. Yet, as sociologist Maren Klawiter has pointed out in her study of breast cancer activism, advocacy and social movements need not necessarily be antagonistic to professional spheres. Instead, she argues, social movements may draw from different social resources and identities, forming specific 'cultures of action' that collaborate or conflict with professionals depending on the situation.[83] Genetics offers good examples for this bandwidth. The NYSPI project relied on developing services in collaboration with local deaf organizations. Parents of children with intellectual disabilities, Alexandra Stern has shown, challenged geneticists' portrayal of the disabled child as a tragedy, yet also relied on them as mediators providing access to other professional services. And Huntington's disease patients and their families explicitly sought to engage scientists in searching for a genetic test and perhaps a cure, contributing their skills and time for these goals.[84]

With Usher syndrome, too, increasingly self-confident advocates challenged the perspectives of mostly hearing-sighted and (increasingly) deaf professionals. They drew inspiration from Deaf and disability activism, but also from the growing professional literature on Usher syndrome and deaf-blindness, which they in turn influenced. Their assertions of self-worth and ability sometimes stood in stark contrast with the perspectives of non-affected professionals. All in all, however, Usher syndrome advocates considered professionals their allies for improving their social, professional, and medical situation. Both sides found common ground in pointing to the harmful effects of bias, exclusion, and discrimination, and to the need to improve the social, educational, and professional situation.

Conclusion

Between the mid-1960s and the mid-1980s, the definition of Usher syndrome and the lives of those affected changed significantly: in the 1960s, it had emerged as a distinguishable condition only because of advances in genetic deafness research. A growing body of knowledge on syndromic forms now marked deaf people as a group at risk for various other conditions, including deaf-blindness. In the following two decades, Usher syndrome went from an obscure, hardly known type of deaf-blindness to being defined as a severely limiting, hereditary, neuro-psychiatric condition, and finally as a progressive sensory disability that carried the risk for psycho-emotional disturbance, yet also the potential for a fulfilled and independent life. This development moved along two narrative arcs that reflected diversifying professional paradigms, changing perceptions of deaf and deaf-blind people, and, not least, larger changes in framing genetic conditions.

One strand of the story rested on the declared need to prevent future misery and suffering. Here Usher syndrome was portrayed as a pressing issue of public health, a matter of economic cost and savings. This narrative arose in the late 1960s from the confluence of older eugenic-medical motives and new attention to neglected minorities and neglected diseases. The expansion of psychiatric and rehabilitation services in the 1950s and 1960s brought attention to deaf-blind patients, forgotten and institutionalized in asylums and psychiatric hospitals. Their condition brought about questions of what exactly Usher syndrome entailed, and what side effects should be expected with a dual sensory deprivation. This relative obscurity allowed Vernon to define Usher syndrome as a hereditary, psycho-neurological condition, connected to a supposed brain lesion that caused not only hearing and vision loss, but also more or less severe psychiatric disturbances. This definition was possible only because it resonated with several larger, connected preconceptions: of severe disability as individual suffering and economic loss for society; of individuals with Usher syndrome as intellectually delayed, mentally disturbed, and unable to care for themselves; and of the unquestioned authority of professionals in defining their condition and status.

With these beliefs in mind, Vernon launched, in the late 1960s, his awareness campaign. It focused on eugenic prevention, and considered improving the lives of individuals with Usher syndrome only a secondary goal at best, even a waste of resources. Prevention, if not eradication, was to be achieved through screening of school-aged children and genetic counselling for their families. Vernon's idea of genetic counselling was directive: individuals' wishes counted little and they were considered ignorant or irresponsible if going against expert recommendations. Perhaps ironically, it was geneticists who tempered overly ambitious hopes for eugenic prevention and eradication. In genetics, such an authoritative stance was no longer in vogue. By the 1970s, geneticists relativized the effects of large-scale screening and prevention on public health, and instead pointed to the emotional benefits of genetic self-awareness. In this sense, the goal of genetic counselling could be to prevent a condition or to provide a first step in preparing to live with it.

This psychologized approach to genetics and disability appealed to different groups. In the 1970s and 1980s, growing awareness of Usher syndrome occurred within a framework of increasingly visible and assertive patient advocacy, disability and Deaf activism, and of professional identification or involvement in such activism. In the interaction between affected individuals, family members, advocates, and professionals there emerged a new image of the individual with Usher syndrome. Rather than helpless and hopeless, isolated or institutionalized patients, they were ordinary people with hopes and plans, families and careers, asserting their continued right to participate in ordinary life.

A second, more recent narrative thus cast Usher syndrome as a journey to self-awareness and self-acceptance. Depending on the perspective, this narrative could take different turns. Physicians, psychologists, teachers, and rehabilitation specialists emphasized the emotional risk faced by individuals with Usher syndrome and their families. Prevention, here, primarily meant avoiding or managing emotional damage through constant professional guidance and surveillance. By the 1980s, Usher syndrome thus had become a psychological as much as a genetic condition. It was a condition that created stress and emotional upheaval for everyone involved: the individual who had to come to terms with a different future; the family, which was dealing with feelings of guilt and anxiety; and not least professionals who had unconscious fears and biases about dealing with deaf-blind individuals. These complicated emotions, professionals asserted, needed to be brought out into the open and dealt with in order to develop appropriate coping mechanisms.

Advocates such as Roehrig and Annala also emphasized the emotional and social impact of becoming deaf-blind, yet portrayed it as a change to adapt to rather than as an end point. Rather than focusing on deficits, they emphasized their strengths, capabilities, and ordinary humanness. They supported the drive for prevention, yet gave primacy to improving access to education and rehabilitation, to addressing bias and exclusion. Drawing from Deaf and disability activism, in particular from the independent living movement, they emphasized their right to a self-determined life. Tapping into the larger social occupation with realizing selfhood, they relativized and normalized Usher syndrome as one life challenge among others. With its emphasis on mastering difficulties and transforming bias and discrimination, this narrative had a strongly empowering dimension.

Genetics, too, could be deployed for a less pathologizing portrayal of Usher syndrome. Geneticists had long emphasized that genetic awareness was an important part of one's self-knowledge, and had carefully observed their clients' emotional coping. For Arthur Roehrig, this notion of genetic awareness resonated with a vision of Usher syndrome as a journey to more profound self-knowledge and self-acceptance. Roehrig took from genetic discourse the often-repeated mantra that one was not at fault for having faulty genes, and that genetic conditions were something that could affect everyone. It was, he argued, part of human variation and difference. This was a notion of genetics that was at once relativizing, and, by making genetics part of one's identity, essentialist. Genetic discourse here was not exclusively an expert conversation that reinforced the ideal – 'healthy' and 'normal' – body. It could also be mobilized for making a case for human diversity – as, indeed, some geneticists had begun doing.

Such overlapping negotiations of disease and disability, physical and emotional risks, professional authority and client autonomy, make Usher syndrome emblematic for larger developments in genetics and deafness research. It makes visible debates over what it meant to have a genetic condition, and how cost-saving measures of eugenic prevention were pitted against the cost of education and rehabilitation – a faulty argument still too common in current discussions of disability and public health. In particular, the history of Usher syndrome also contributes to the lesser-explored zone between the histories of science and medicine, deafness, disability, and activism, which will be further explored in the next chapter.

Notes

1. M. Vernon, 'Usher's syndrome – deafness and progressive blindness: clinical cases, prevention, theory and literature survey', *Journal of Chronic Diseases*, 22:3 (1969), 133–51.
2. Such estimates always depend on the population in question, and are also relative to the changing frequency of other causes of deafness. For current estimates see National Institute on Deafness and Other Communication Disorders, 'Usher Syndrome', NIDCD Fact Sheet, www.nidcd.nih.gov/health/hearing/pages/usher.aspx#b [accessed 25 September 2018]. Current research distinguishes between three different forms of Usher syndrome: Type 1 and 2, in which profound or moderate hearing loss is present at birth, and vision loss begins in adolescence, and Type 3, in which vision and hearing loss begins in adolescence. These distinctions had not yet been made in the period this chapter is covering.
3. See e.g. S. N. Barnartt and R. K. Scotch, *Disability Protests: Contentious Politics 1970–1999* (Washington, DC: Gallaudet University Press, 2001); D. Zames Fleischer and F. Zames, *The Disability Rights Movement: From Charity to Confrontation* (Philadelphia, PA: Temple University Press, 2011); K. Jankowski, *Deaf Empowerment: Emergence, Struggle, and Rhetoric* (Washington, DC: Gallaudet University Press, 2013).
4. See e.g. M. Vernon and W. Hicks, 'A group counseling and educational program for students with Usher's syndrome', *Journal of Visual Impairment and Blindness*, 77:2 (1983), 64–6.
5. See C. Rocheleau and R. Mack, *Those in Dark Silence: The Deaf-Blind in North America; a Record of To-Day* (Washington, DC: The Volta Bureau, 1930). For a critique of such stereotyping see e.g. J. Miele Rodas, 'On blindness', *Journal of Cultural and Literary Disability Studies*, 3:2 (2009), 115–20.
6. (Auto)biographies of famous deaf-blind people give a limited insight. See e.g. K. E. Nielsen, *The Radical Lives of Helen Keller* (New York: New York University Press, 2009). For an activist perspective, see J. L. Clark, *Where I Stand: On the Signing Community and My Deafblind Experience* (Minneapolis, MN: Handtype Press, 2014). For the emergence of the pro-tactile movement see the work of Terra Edwards, e.g. T. Edwards, 'Language emergence in the Seattle DeafBlind community' (PhD dissertation, University of California, 2014).
7. See e.g. M. Vernon, 'Overview of Usher's syndrome: congenital deafness and progressive loss of vision', *The Volta Review*, 76:2 (1974), 100–5.
8. See C. H. Usher, 'On the inheritance of retinitis pigmentosa, with notes of cases', *Royal London Ophthalmic Hospital Reports*, 19 (1914), 122–236.
9. See e.g. H. W. Kloepfer, J. K. Laguaite, and J. W. Mclaurin, 'The hereditary syndrome of congenital deafness and retinitis pigmentosa (Usher's syndrome)', *The Laryngoscope*, 76:5 (1966), 850–62.
10. Gallaudet University Archives, MSS 048, Vernon, McCay, Box 5, Folder 23,

McCay Vernon, correspondence 'Usher syndrome' (1966–1974), 'Vernon to Ian Shine', 15 March 1967.
11 See the informational film produced by Vernon and colleagues, M. Vernon, L. E. Griswold, and Gallaudet College, *Usher's Syndrome: Retinitis Pigmentosa and Deafness* (Washington DC: Gallaudet College, 1978).
12 Vernon, 'Usher's syndrome'.
13 R. S. Grinker, 'Foreword', in Grinker (ed.), *Psychiatric Diagnosis*, pp. 8–11, here p. 8.
14 *Ibid.*
15 *Ibid.*
16 M. Vernon, *Multiply Handicapped Deaf Children: Medical, Educational, and Psychological Considerations* (Washington, DC: Council for Exceptional Children, 1969).
17 Grinker, *Psychiatric Diagnosis*, p. 9.
18 Schlesinger, 'Cultural and environmental influences', p. 131.
19 M. Vernon and B. Makowsky, 'Deafness and minority group dynamics: sociological and psychological factors associated with hearing loss', *The Deaf American*, 21:11 (1963), 3–6, here 3–5.
20 *Ibid.*, 6. For the history of the model minority myth see e.g. E. D. Wu, *Color of Success – Asian Americans and the Origins of the Model Minority* (Princeton, NJ: Princeton University Press, 2015).
21 M. Vernon, 'The final report', in Grinker (ed.), *Psychiatric Diagnosis*, pp. 13–37, here pp. 15–16.
22 H. Lane, 'Cochlear implants: their cultural and historical meaning', in J. V. Van Cleve (ed.), *Deaf History Unveiled: Interpretations from the New Scholarship* (Washington, DC: Gallaudet University Press, 1993), pp. 273–91, here p. 280.
23 See Burch, *Signs of Resistance*, pp. 2–5; Robinson, '"We are a different class"'.
24 For a discussion of deaf-blindness and psychopathology see e.g. S. B. Wortis and D. Shaskan, 'Retinitis Pigmentosa and associated neuropsychiatric changes', *The Journal of Nervous and Mental Disease*, 92:4 (1940), 1990–1; B. Hallgren, 'Retinitis pigmentosa in combination with congenital deafness and vestibulocerebellar ataxia; with psychiatric abnormality in some cases; a clinical and genetic study', *Acta Genetica Et Statistica Medica*, 8:2 (1958), 97–104; J. G. Small and G. M. Desmarais, 'The familial occurrence of retinitis pigmentosa, mental disorders and EEG abnormalities', *The American Journal of Psychiatry*, 122:11 (1966), 1286–9.
25 Vernon, 'Usher's syndrome – deafness and progressive blindness', 145.
26 *Ibid.*, 140.
27 M. Vernon, 'Usher's syndrome: problems and some solutions', *Hearing and Speech Action*, 44:4 (1976), 6–7, 9–13, here 9.
28 *Ibid.*, 9, 11.
29 See e.g. S. A. Plotkin, 'The history of rubella and rubella vaccination leading to elimination', *Clinical Infectious Diseases: An Official Publication of the Infectious Diseases Society of America*, 43 (2005), 164–8.

30 In part, these widely varying estimations were due to shifting definitions about the degree of visual and auditory impairment constituting deaf-blindness. By the mid-1980s some estimated that only 800 individuals were affected by rubella-caused deaf-blindness. See e.g. E. R. Stuckless, 'Rubella and the human burden', in E. M. Gruenberg, C. Lewis, and S. E. Goldston (eds), *Vaccinating Against Brain Syndromes: The Campaign Against Measles and Rubella* (New York: Oxford University Press, 1986), pp. 70–9.
31 See L. J. Reagan, *Dangerous Pregnancies: Mothers, Disabilities, and Abortion in America* (Berkeley, CA: University of California Press, 2010), pp. 1, 4, 222.
32 For this development see e.g. J. D. Schein, 'A brief history of services for deafblind people in the US', in C. L. Graham (ed.), *Transition Planning for Students Who Are DeafBlind* (Knoxville, TN: PEPNet-South, 2007), pp. 7–19; G. D. Brewer and J. S. Kakalis, *Serving the Deaf-Blind Population: Planning for 1980* (Santa Monica, CA: Rand Corp, 1974), p. 1.
33 See e.g. Stuckless, 'Rubella and the human burden'.
34 Vernon, 'Overview of Usher's syndrome', 100.
35 Brewer and Kalikakis, *Serving the Deaf-Blind*, p. 10.
36 Reagan, *Dangerous Pregnancies*, p. 8.
37 Plotkin, 'History of rubella', 165–6.
38 For the history of PKU see D. B. Paul and J. P. Brosco, *The PUK Paradox: A Short History of a Genetic Disease* (Baltimore, MD: Johns Hopkins University Press, 2014).
39 See e.g. Vernon, 'Overview of Usher's syndrome'.
40 Gallaudet University Archives, MSS 048, Vernon, McCay, Box 5, Folder 22, McCay Vernon, correspondence 'Usher syndrome' (1966–1974).
41 Ibid.
42 Vernon, 'Overview of Usher's syndrome', 102.
43 See Wailoo, *Dying in the City of the Blues*; Wailoo and Pemberton, *The Troubled Dream of Genetic Medicine*.
44 C. W. Day, 'Current screening procedures for the Usher syndrome at residential schools for the deaf', *American Annals of the Deaf*, 127:1 (1982), 45–8.
45 E. Hammer, 'Needs of adolescents who have Usher's Syndrome', *American Annals of the Deaf*, 123:3 (1978), 389–94, here 389.
46 M. Vernon, J. A. Boughman, and L. Annala, 'Considerations in diagnosing Usher's syndrome: RP and hearing loss', *Journal of Visual Impairment and Blindness*, 76:7 (1982), 258–61, here 259–60.
47 For different positions see e.g. Hammer, 'Needs of adolescents', 393; Day, 'Current screening procedures', 45; A. Roehrig, 'Living with Usher's syndrome', in N. L. Tully (ed.), *Papers Presented at a Workshop on Usher's Syndrome, December 2–3, 1976. Conducted by Helen Keller National Center for Deaf-Blind Youths and Adults* (Sands Point, NY: Helen Keller National Center, 1977), pp. 23–7, here p. 26; Vernon and Hicks, 'A group counseling and educational program', 64.
48 C. Torrie, 'Families with adolescent children with Usher's Syndrome: developing

services to meet their needs', *American Annals of the Deaf*, special edition, 'Usher's syndrome: the personal, social, and emotional implication', ed. J. English, 123:3 (1978), 359–420, here 382, 385, 387–8.
49 *Ibid.*, p. 385.
50 W. Nance, 'Genetic aspects of Usher's syndrome', in *Symposium on Usher's Syndrome, Washington, D. C., April 19, 1973* (Washington, DC: Public Service Programs, Gallaudet College, 1973), pp. 12–18, here pp. 15–17. Also see W. Nance, Walter, J. B. Campbell, and F. R. Bieber, 'The Usher syndrome: a long neglected genetic disease', in Tully (ed.), *Workshop on Usher's Syndrome*, pp. 4–7.
51 M. J. E. Harrod, 'Genetic counseling for Usher's syndrome patients and their families', in Tully (ed.), *Workshop on Usher's Syndrome*, pp. 376–80, here pp. 377–9.
52 *Ibid.*
53 In 2017, Gallaudet University established a scholarship for deaf-blind students in Annala's honour. See A. Talaat, 'The Linda Annala, '70, scholarship', *Gallaudet University News*, 3 April 2017, www.gallaudet.edu/news/linda-annala-scholarship-fund [7 October 2018].
54 L. Annala, 'Facing the future with Usher syndrome', in Tully (ed.), *Workshop on Usher's Syndrome*, pp. 19–22, here p. 19.
55 *Ibid.*, pp. 19–20.
56 *Ibid.*, p. 20.
57 *Ibid.*
58 A. Roehrig, 'Coping with the discovery of Usher's syndrome', in *Symposium on Usher's Syndrome*, pp. 32–8, here pp. 34–5.
59 *Ibid.*, pp. 32, 36.
60 *Ibid.*, pp. 36–7.
61 For the interest in the self and in self-help see e.g. G. Eghigian, A. Killen, and C. Leuenberger (eds), *The Self as Project: Politics and the Human Sciences* (Chicago, IL: University of Chicago Press, 2007); N. Rose, *Governing the Soul: The Shaping of the Private Self* (London: Routledge, 1990).
62 M. M. Lock and V.-K. Nguyen, *An Anthropology of Biomedicine* (Chichester, West Sussex: Wiley-Blackwell, 2010), pp. 283, 298, 301.
63 See e.g. E. Goffman, *Stigma Notes on the Management of Spoiled Identity* (Englewood Cliffs, NJ: Prentice-Hall, 1963); I. K. Zola, 'Helping one another: a speculative history of the self-help movement', *Archives of Physical Medicine and Rehabilitation*, 60:10 (1979), 452–6; I. K. Zola, *Missing Pieces: A Chronicle of Living with a Disability* (Philadelphia, PA: Temple University Press, 1982).
64 W. E. Nance, *What Every Person Should Know about Heredity and Deafness* (Washington, DC: Gallaudet College, 1975), p. 1.
65 *Ibid.*, p. 26.
66 Roehrig, 'Living with Usher's syndrome', p. 25.
67 See e.g. A. Wexler, *Mapping Fate: A Memoir of Family, Risk, and Genetic Research* (New York: Times Books, 1995); S. M. Lindee, 'Genetic disease in the 1960s: a structural revolution', *American Journal of Medical Genetics*, 115:2 (2002),

75–82; S. M. Lindee, *Moments of Truth in Genetic Medicine* (Baltimore, MD: Johns Hopkins University Press, 2005); A. E. Raz, *Community Genetics and Genetic Alliances: Eugenics, Carrier Testing and Networks of Risk* (London: Routledge, 2010).
68 Annala, 'Facing the future', pp. 19, 20, 22.
69 Roehrig, 'Living with Usher's syndrome', pp. 23, 25.
70 Annala, 'Facing the future', pp. 21, 22.
71 *Ibid.*
72 A. Pimentel, 'Handling the upper secondary and college Usher's syndrome student', in Tully, *Workshop on Usher's Syndrome*, pp. 51–6, here pp. 51–2.
73 *Ibid.*
74 Roehrig, 'Coping with the discovery of Usher's syndrome', p. 32.
75 Roehrig, 'Living with Usher's syndrome', pp. 24–5.
76 *Ibid.*, p. 26.
77 See e.g. L. Patterson, 'Points of access: rehabilitation centers, summer camps, and student life in the making of disability activism, 1960–1973', *Journal of Social History*, 46:2 (2012), 473–99.
78 See e.g. Zola, 'Helping one another'. Also see C. Barnes and G. Mercer, *Independent Futures: Creating User-Led Disability Services in a Disabling Society* (Bristol: Policy Press, 2006), pp. 29–49.
79 Roehrig, 'Living with Usher's syndrome', p. 36.
80 Patterson, 'Points of access', 472–3.
81 Jankowski, *Deaf Empowerment*, p. 94. For a similar position, see Zames Fleischer and Zames, *Disability Rights Movements*, pp. 15–32. For a more nuanced discussion of the commonalities and differences see Burch and Kafer, *Deaf and Disability Studies*; Padden, 'Talking culture'.
82 Such multiple and overlapping deaf identities are a growing field for research. See e.g. H D. Clark, 'We are the same but different: navigating African American and deaf cultural identities' (PhD dissertation, University of Washington, 2010); A. Werner, '"Double whammy"?! Historical glimpses of black deaf Americans', *COPAS*, 18:2 (2017), https://copas.uni-regensburg.de/article/view/288 [accessed 10 October 2019].
83 M. Klawiter, *The Biopolitics of Breast Cancer: Changing Cultures of Disease and Activism* (Minneapolis, MN: University of Minnesota Press, 2008), pp. 44, 134.
84 Stern, *Telling Genes*, pp. 77–97; Wexler, *Mapping Fate*.

5

SIGNING RISK AND CHANCE: COLLABORATING FOR CULTURALLY SENSITIVE COUNSELLING, 1970–1990

In the early 1970s, geneticist Walter Nance counselled a deaf couple on their risk of having a deaf child. For Nance, this was a standard procedure. The couple's reaction, however, made him question his approach and beliefs. 'It is a sobering experience', he recalled later, 'to spend an hour communicating the facts of genetics to a deaf couple through an interpreter, only to be confronted by the question from the shy young bride, "What is wrong with being deaf?"'[1] What, indeed, was wrong with it? If one believed in genetics as a science that served the individual rather than society, in client autonomy and non-directiveness, there was no longer a normative answer to this question. Rather, Nance believed, geneticists should learn about deaf people's needs and preferences.

Once more, this chapter looks at what happened when scientists came into contact with deaf people whose beliefs challenged their own. In a way, such encounters had been a constant in hereditary deafness research, and more generally in the interaction between hearing and deaf people. Reactions were, and still are, determined by preconceptions and polarized perspectives, by what and where someone first learned about deafness and who deaf people should be. Sometimes, however, an encounter between hearing and deaf perspectives was startling or jarring enough to trigger a curiosity to learn more. During the first half of the twentieth century this was easier said than done. There were no sign language classes or books about deaf culture or community. Professional literature almost uniformly defined deafness as a defect and deaf people as somewhat defective. Professional associations were strictly hearing, and in any case, scientists and physicians carefully maintained the line between themselves and lay people. This had changed by the early 1970s. Support for sign language or bilingual approaches had been growing rapidly, as had linguistic and sociological research into Deaf culture and community. This did little to ease the old polarization and animosity between supporters of oralism and sign language, but it had a snowballing effect that made a cultural model of deafness available and imaginable for someone like Nance. The old lines between hearing professionals and deaf service recipients was weakening, too. For professionals, it had become attractive to associate oneself with activists and social movements campaigning for social justice or equality in health care.

As a physician and geneticist, Nance had learned to think about deafness as a pathology to be cured and prevented. Yet his encounters with signing deaf clients and their values triggered a reorientation, one that he tried to apply in a more culturally sensitive form of genetic counselling. Over the next two decades, he worked with this as his goal with two of his students and future colleagues, Joann Boughman and Kathleen Shaver Arnos. They believed that in order to provide genetic services to deaf people, they first had to learn about their culture, values, and language. For Boughman and Arnos, in particular, this meant learning sign language and trying to assimilate to Deaf culture. In turn, counselling in sign language sensitized them for different perceptions of genetic risk and to the bias inherent in genetic terminology. Engaging with their deaf clients and surrounding communities, they negotiated the disconnection between a medical-genetic community, which considered deafness a pathology to be cured and prevented, and the Deaf community, which considered deafness the distinguishing trait of their community. Throughout the 1970s and 1980s, they became involved in the emerging Usher syndrome community, conducted research on genetics and rubella, and developed ASL signs for genetic counselling. These projects culminated in the establishment of a Genetic Services Center at Gallaudet in 1984. Referring to deaf people's minority rights and cultural identity, the centre operated within an increasingly diversified and politicized arena of deafness and disability, health care and health care activism. Promoting genetic self-awareness as an important part of individual identity and political empowerment, it actively took part in this politicisation – and, I argue, helped prepare a biology-based identity politics in Deaf activism.

Counselling the deaf – or being counselled by the deaf?

'No single group', Walter Nance claimed in 1971, 'can profit more from [genetic] counseling than the hearing impaired'.[2] It was, he believed, 'one universally applicable form of therapy for hereditary deafness'.[3] In the history of genetics, the profits gained from genetic information have been defined in different ways: genetic counselling can inform the individual, couple, or family about their risk for a certain hereditary trait, and thus act as a form of disease prevention. For most of the twentieth century, this medical-eugenic paradigm was the main reason for seeking or providing genetic information. It probably is still foremost on people's minds when they seek genetic counselling. For Nance, too, recent progress in identifying the biochemical bases of genetic deafness held great promise. 'Here, truly', he wrote with the unrealized enthusiasm typical within genetics, 'we have a cure looking for a disease'.[4] Yet from mid-century on, geneticists also increasingly emphasized the emotional and psychological benefits of genetic awareness, and thus, implicitly, of being prepared for the future.

As a physician turned geneticist, Nance was familiar both with genetic counselling as a means of disease prevention, and as an instrument for providing advice and emotional support. Over the course of the 1970s, he not only came to emphasize more the psychosocial benefits of genetic counselling, he also developed a more relative definition of deafness, no longer automatically assuming it was something to be cured or prevented. On the contrary, he believed that if a deaf couple wished to have a deaf child, the geneticist might well be able and willing to assist them in realizing this wish. This reorientation was influenced by encounters with deaf people and Deaf culture, and was embedded in larger debates over non-directiveness and patient autonomy in genetic counselling.

Certainly, his personality and personal background played a role too. Born in Manila in 1933 to the family of an American surgeon, he was early on exposed to different cultures and languages, and had personal experiences with disability. During his childhood, the family first moved to Shanghai, then, with the 1941 evacuation of all American civilians from China, back to the US. Living in New Orleans, Nance, aged twelve or thirteen, contracted polio after swimming in the Mississippi. His left arm was left paralysed, although he later regained some mobility. Like many in the polio generation, he was taught not to think of his paralysed arm as a disability. In 1954, he entered Harvard Medical School after graduating with a BA from the University of the South in Sewanee.[5] While he was in college, his parents had another child, his brother Benji; 'the sibling', he believes, 'that arguably has had the most influence on my life'. At birth, the obstetrician diagnosed Benji with Down syndrome. Benji, Nance recalled, 'was one of the most severely affected infants with Down syndrome I've ever seen', never learning to sit or walk. Like many intellectually disabled children of his generation, Nance's brother lived not at home, but first in a private nursing home, then in a public facility, where he died of a respiratory infection at age ten.[6]

Benji's life and early death, and his parents' search for support and therapy triggered Nance's interest in medicine, and his fascination with genetics.

Patients with a family history of certain conditions reinforced this fascination. Twin studies, in particular, caught his interest and became a lifelong research focus. After graduating from Harvard in 1958, Nance began his residency in internal medicine at Vanderbilt University. Among his colleagues, he soon 'got a reputation ... of being more interested in the family history than the present illness'.[7] His chairman, David Rogers (son of famous therapist Carl Rogers), jokingly suggested one day, "'Walter, maybe you better go study genetics before you hurt somebody'".[8]

From 1961 to 1968, Nance pursued his PhD in genetics at the University of Madison, Wisconsin Department of Genetics, led by distinguished geneticist James F. Crow. From 1963 on, he combined his PhD research with a position as assistant professor of medicine and head of the division of medical genetics at the Vanderbilt University School of Medicine. Simultaneously seeing patients at Vanderbilt and studying biochemical genetics in Madison intensified Nance's interest in defining genetic conditions at the clinical and the molecular level. One of these conditions was deafness. He first encountered a deaf patient with a family history of hearing loss in the late 1960s. Intrigued, he visited the patient's family in a very rural part of southwestern Tennessee. The patient, he learned there, 'was a product of a first-cousin marriage'. This made heredity a likely cause, and alerted Nance to the existence of pedigree data collected outside of the clinic. His realization led him to the Tennessee School for the Deaf in Knoxville, where generations of deaf students had generated rich records.[9]

Nance's first forays into genetic deafness research soon found an institutional context in Nashville's Bill Wilkerson Hearing and Speech Center. Established in 1951 by otolaryngologist Wesley Wilkerson, it provided speech training and medical services to deaf children and researched hearing loss. In particular, the centre offered services to toddlers and pre-schoolers, a group few schools served at the time. To their parents, the centre offered the promise that deafness was a fixable disability, if only professionals, parents, and the child tried hard enough, and if only the child was reached by spoken language as early as possible. The centre thus was part of a longer tradition of scientific oralism that promised the deaf child's eventual normalization through ever more advanced medical-technological intervention. Recent advances in individual hearing aid technology spurred this belief. Consequently, the Wilkerson Center purposefully put hearing before speech, both in their name and in their daily work. Their own research was to further this goal. Most research took place in audiology or speech therapy, yet genetic deafness research and counselling, too, was included.[10] Nance was part of the interdisciplinary Vanderbilt Hereditary Deafness Group, which came together in a weekly clinic to discuss cases and provide genetic counselling to families with suspected hereditary deafness. Supported by a Department of Health, Education, and Welfare grant, the group also conducted genetic research in rural Tennessee.[11]

At the Wilkerson Clinic and at Vanderbilt, Nance thus began his research in a setting that defined deafness firmly as a pathology to be identified, cured, ameliorated, or prevented. Genetics fitted seamlessly into this larger mission. Parents and their hearing-impaired children came to the centre for audiological services or speech therapy, and, once there, learnt about yet another, potentially intergenerational dimension of hearing loss. In this institutional context, Nance's early deafness research remained distant and abstract explorations of pedigrees and biochemical phenomena. Soon, however, he encountered more probing deaf perspectives that questioned his own.

Coming across Edgar Allen Fay's 1898 *Marriages of the Deaf in America*, he immediately realized the value of Fay's tabulated pedigree information for current research.[12] Most of this material was housed at Gallaudet. Gallaudet – long the academic and social centre of American Deaf culture – presented Nance with a very different image of deafness and deaf people. In the 1970s and 1980s, the campus and more generally the DC area, with its strong network of well-educated students and alumni, became the most visible centre of a new kind of Deaf activism.[13] Visiting Gallaudet for his research, and being 'thoroughly exposed to a large number of individuals who were communicating in sign language', left 'a strong impression' with Nance. He commented: 'I realized that if this was going to be a major interest of mine that I needed to know about and hopefully embrace the attitudes of the deaf towards their hearing loss'.[14]

Nance began collaborating with Gallaudet during the 1970s, at a time when it transformed from a small, isolated liberal arts college into a modern research university and centre of academic research on Deaf culture.[15] Working with Gallaudet's Office of Demographic Studies (formerly Offices of Institutional Research and Psychological Research), he helped expand research activity and was exposed to Deaf culture and community. Among the Office's recurrent administrative tasks was the Annual Survey of Deaf and Hard of Hearing Children and Youths, which since 1968 has collected one confidential form per student from all schools serving this group. The results, adding up to the most extensive database of childhood deafness in the US, have been used to plan educational needs and services. Collecting data on family background, aetiology, and onset of deafness, the annual survey also provided valuable information for Nance's genetic research.[16]

Under clinical psychologist Jerome D. Schein, the Office of Demographic Studies had a director well suited for turning current sociopolitical thought into academic research. Schein, who headed the centre from 1966 to 1968, was a hearing, lifelong advocate for the Deaf community and sign languages. His 1968 *The Deaf Community: Studies in the Social Psychology of Deafness*, in some ways replicated the NYSPI survey of the New York State deaf population, to which he referred frequently. Yet in the more politicized and polarized 1970s, Schein more empathetically described deaf people as a sociocultural minority, and vehemently criticized the bias and discrimination affecting them. Deafness, he believed, 'is not a disease, it is a functional disorder' – and it was external factors – professional bias and 'sensory, linguistic, and experiential deprivations' similar to those experienced by black people or other minorities – which often turned it into a disorder in first place.[17]

Exposed to signing deaf people and a deafness-as-culture perspective lived and researched at Gallaudet, Nance reoriented his approach to deafness – and tried to bring his colleagues along. At a 1977 conference on genetic counselling, he explained that some 'deaf individuals do not feel that deafness is a handicap'. This group appeared to be a minority. Nevertheless, their opinion should be accepted: 'I would certainly respect the right of a deaf couple to want a deaf child'. To achieve this end, he continued, the geneticist could even 'help them select a partner'. For Nance, genetics was to be an enabling profession, assisting clients with their reproductive preferences.[18] Genetically informed decision-making, not prevention, was the goal. Genetic knowledge, he believed, was as indispensable for deaf people and their families, as it was for the hearing, if not more so. Yet it was unattainable for most. '[G]enetic counseling of the deaf and for the parents of the deaf', he explained to various audiences in the mid- and late 1970s, was a 'major unmet need'.[19] To meet it, geneticists had to explore and acknowledge deaf people's beliefs, and adapt counselling practice accordingly. Together with two of his students, Nance set out to realize this goal.

From risk to chance: the transformative effect of counselling in sign language

Like Nance, Joann Boughman had not known deaf people before entering genetics, and like Nance, encounters with deaf clients changed her perspectives on deafness and counselling. Her professional coming of age, however, occurred in a time of more politicized and visible Deaf and health care activism.

For the Deaf community, the 1970s were a transitional period of upward mobility and growing visibility. These changes were fostered by new kinds of socializing and activism. Activists engaged in awareness-raising protests or anti-discrimination lawsuits, bringing deaf people to public attention as one of America's minorities striving for equality, acceptance, and access.[20] In this invigorating social climate, Boughman went further than Nance in her identification with and assimilation to the Deaf community. Her encounters with deaf people turned client autonomy and non-directive counselling into practical issues and challenged her beliefs about genetic risk, disability, and counselling.

Graduating from Indiana University with a BS in medical technology (clinical laboratory science) in 1972, Boughman applied and was accepted to the university's PhD programme in medical genetics. Walter Nance, who had left Vanderbilt for a professorship in medical genetics at Indiana University (IU) in 1969, became her advisor. At IU, students of medical genetics received a broad training in basic genetic research and its clinical applications, including courses in probability and statistics, biochemistry, biochemical and population genetics. The last was a field to which Boughman was particularly drawn and remained involved with for the rest of her career. She wrote her PhD thesis on retinitis pigmentosa and became involved with the growing deaf-blind community. Students were also trained in genetic counselling. Approaching the counselling situation as a dynamic process required that the counsellor reflected on his or her emotions and relationship with clients. Consequently, it was important to understand and react to clients' emotions and expectations in relation to their sociocultural and educational background, and to discuss what this meant to non-directive counselling.[21]

Boughman's graduate training fell into a time of professionalization and change in genetic counselling. Most prominently, this change was shaped by the graduates of new MA programmes, who successfully claimed a niche in a field formerly occupied solely by MDs or PhDs. The first of these programmes was established in 1969 at Sarah Lawrence College in Bronxville, New York; others soon followed. The vast majority of graduates were (and remain to this day) women. For them, pursuing a degree in genetic counselling provided an opportunity for a career in health care. Sympathetic to the second wave Women's Movement, these predominantly white middle-class counsellors believed respecting reproductive autonomy was an important part of their professional ethics. Most considered preventing disease and suffering to be an important goal of genetics, yet they also were aware that client goals and values might differ from their own. Moreover, unlike the research-focused PhD or clinically minded MD geneticists, they entered counselling specifically to assist clients in making genetically informed decisions in emotionally challenging situations. In doing so, they tapped into an older tradition of assigning female health care professionals to caring, assisting, and helping roles. Genetic counselling thus became a field associated with 'female' qualities – with the usual implications for pay and status.[22]

Although she chose a more traditional path into genetics, Boughman, too, identified with this ideal of genetic counselling as a nurturing and care-giving profession. Genetics, she later explained, differed from other medical professions in that they could offer empathy and support, but often no medical solutions, much less a cure. Unlike physicians, whose goal it was to 'make people well' or at least 'better', geneticists had never been 'in the fixing business'.[23] It could be 'hard not to', she acknowledged, yet whether it was deafness or rare diseases, geneticists usually dealt with conditions that could not be medically fixed. This was a realistic and humble assessment that was based on geneticists' everyday experience and contrasted with long-standing grander claims about a genetic fix to disease and disability. It affected attitudes towards disability and deafness. Seeing their professional purpose in curing people, Boughman thought, physicians were 'uncomfortable' if this wasn't possible – and 'frustrated' with (deaf) patients who did not want to be cured in first place.[24] As a geneticist, she believed, you 'have to have a different attitude toward ability and the range of ability'. It didn't matter so much at 'what point you call something a *dis*ability' than 'at what point you call things a challenge and try to deal with the challenge'.[25] Here, genetics had 'been pretty good' in referring people 'to the right kind of help and support systems', helping to 'develop networks and so on so that people always had other people to interact with that were living the same kind of challenges'.[26]

Still a graduate student, she soon began to assist Nance on his field trips to schools for the deaf, using her skills as a medical technologist. Here she gained her first counselling experiences. Counselling deaf clients brought new perspectives and insights. On one of these field trips to the Indiana School for the Deaf, for example, they diagnosed a young deaf man with retinitis pigmentosa. Telling him and his family that he had Usher syndrome and would eventually become deaf-blind was a turning point in Boughman's professional life. The fact that, at this point, neither she nor Nance knew sign language, and had to rely on an interpreter added communication insecurity to an already emotionally taxing situation. To Boughman, it 'was an absolutely devastating experience'. Discussing the event with Nance, she decided to learn sign language herself.[27] Only by eliminating the intermediary position of the interpreter, she believed, would the counsellor be able to react immediately and without distortion to clients' emotions, questions, and fears.

By the 1970s, it had become quite common for hearing people to take sign language classes, for a variety of professional or personal reasons. Signing Deaf artists, actors, and activists entered mainstream art and media, as a new appreciation for physical expressivity in pop and counter cultures replaced older negative attitudes. Most prominently, perhaps, the National Theatre of the Deaf, founded in 1967 by deaf actors with the support of Edna Levine and Boyce Williams, made ASL visible as a language of the fine arts on stages and TV screens all over the US. In this politicized atmosphere, learning sign language meant coming into contact with a group that was asserting its role in a more diverse American society.[28]

For Boughman, taking classes and becoming 'relatively fluent in sign' proved to be a transformative experience. It triggered an interest in learning more about Deaf culture, initiated her to the Deaf community, and opened new venues for counselling deaf clients. 'It was kind of like the ocean', she described her experience, 'first it's small waves and then it just kind of consumes you'. She began attending activities organized by Richmond Deaf clubs, and served as a reverse interpreter and as a member of the board of directors of the Commonwealth Theatre of the Deaf in Virginia. Through her work on deaf-blindness, she got to know Arthur Roehrig and got involved in the Washington Area Club for the Deaf-Blind. In her counselling, even though she still used an interpreter when needed, she now was able to communicate and interact more directly with deaf clients.[29]

Learning and operating in a different language makes one aware that translation is often just an approximation, that words and concepts in one language do not match perfectly with those from another. For Boughman, counselling in sign language brought the realization that this was true for 'risk', too. It was a relative concept, depending on client experience and background. As a population geneticist, she thought of risk as an abstract, statistical entity that she and her colleagues calculated from pedigrees and population data. Geneticists use different forms of risk assessment, depending on the data available. The study of genetic risk had greatly expanded after World War II, particularly from the 1960s on. Advances in cyto- and biochemical genetics and computational biology allowed for more precise, individualized predictions. Increasingly, assessing genetic risk became a highly complex biostatistics enterprise, requiring a high level of expertise. The vast majority of counselling clients, on the other hand, were neither familiar with statistics nor with biomedicine, and, as Boughman observed, often had a quiet different understanding of risk. She was not alone in this observation. From the 1970s on, research on the social dimensions of risk perception helped geneticists understand why for some clients a risk of 10, 25, or 50 per cent was significant, while for others it was acceptable or negligible.[30]

Boughman's deaf clients, however, not only had a different perception of numerical risk, they also questioned what counted as risk or defect in the first place. One counselling session in the late 1970s in particular demonstrated this. As she explained to a deaf couple their 'risk' of having a deaf child, the husband, she recounted, 'said [signed] stop'. Explaining the difficulties of raising a hearing child, the prospective father signed, 'we don't want to know the risk of a deaf child, we want to know the risk of a hearing child'. At 'that moment', she recalled, 'my entire perspective was reversed'.[31] Counselling in English, she had often used 'risk' and 'chance' interchangeably. Confronted with the corresponding signs, the visual impression of the 'the closed fist [risk] and the open hand [chance]' drastically visualized 'the difference in the concepts'. This experience changed her counselling practice and terminology not only with deafness, but 'in all other counseling situations as well': from 'that time on, I didn't use the word risk, I used chance'.[32] Retold as a conversation between equals, this counselling session placed the authority to define deafness in the hands – literally – of those with lived experience rather than with the medical professional.

Boughman's reconceptualization of genetic risk occurred alongside a redefinition of deafness as being on the normal end of the hearing-not-hearing dichotomy. Sign language, rather than English, served as the vehicle for this change, signalling the expert's willingness to assimilate to client culture. The counselling session had turned into a 'two-way learning experience'. It made Boughman dependent on and indebted to her clients' willingness to share their values and beliefs. She explained: 'I will be forever grateful to that couple in that moment, because it really did change me'. Her 'genetic counseling experiences', she explained, 'helped formulate and define my understanding and feelings about [...] deaf culture and appreciate their position'.[33] Her admiration for ASL as an effective and beautiful language signalled closeness and identification rather than scientific distance or superiority on part of the hearing geneticist.

In the following years, Boughman put herself in the role of a cultural ambassador between the Deaf and the genetics communities. She shared her experiences with her colleagues at the Indiana University Department of Genetics, a group frequently engaged in discussions about counselling terminology, and invited them to watch counselling sessions in sign language. Observing such sessions was a particularly powerful way to convey the difference between sessions with and without an interpreter, of direct and mediated communication. Sign language, she believed, 'is so beautiful and so expressive that they ... could appreciate it even if they didn't know how to sign'. Because of its visual qualities, she considered ASL better suited than English to explain the difference between the abstract concepts of 'risk' and 'chance' – a belief that contrasted sharply with the long-held belief that sign languages cannot convey abstractions.[34]

Research on and counselling for genetic deafness, Boughman became convinced, should be a cooperative enterprise with input from both geneticists and the Deaf community. This required the geneticists not only to learn about Deaf culture (as Nance had done), but to become an accepted part of it, to assimilate.

A 'small supportive culture': fieldwork and immersion

In the 1980s, Boughman pursued a number of projects together with Nance and their PhD student and future colleague, Kathleen Shaver Arnos, who was also intensely interested in using sign language to provide culturally sensitive genetic counselling. Unlike Nance and Boughman, who had come to deafness via genetics, Arnos came to genetics via a BA in psychology. Yet she, too, had always been interested in basic science, enough to begin her undergraduate career at Western Maryland College (now McDaniel College) majoring in biology and chemistry. Psychology classes provided Arnos with a first contact with deaf people and Deaf culture, and to influential advocates such as McCay Vernon, who spent most of his career as a professor of psychology at Western Maryland. In the 1970s, the college became a centre of deaf graduate education. Its pioneering Master's programme in deaf education, established in 1967, used a total communication approach that used both ASL and English. At a time in which deaf people still faced massive barriers in higher education, it explicitly accepted deaf students, and drew a cadre of motivated young deaf professionals, who brought with them their beliefs about Deaf culture and community.[35] Arnos sat in Vernon's classes, which were taught simultaneously in English and ASL; an experience that motivated her to take sign language classes herself.[36]

Vernon and Arnos, it turned out, shared an interest in genetics, psychology and deafness. He introduced her to Walter Nance, now at the Medical College of Virginia (MCV) in Richmond. In 1979, Arnos was accepted to its PhD programme in human genetics, which she entered with a specific goal in mind: Vernon had sensitized her to the 'great need ... for someone who is fluent' in ASL and encouraged her to become 'the first genetic counselor who works in the deaf community'.[37] With Nance and Boughman, she found advisors strongly supportive of this goal. Boughman and Arnos in particular bonded over their shared love for sign language and Deaf culture. Boughman welcomed the arrival of a person with whom she could practise sign language. 'Kathy and I', she recalled, 'would sign to each other and drive everyone around us crazy'. They 'stimulated each other's interest in absorbing the culture and jumping in'. Nance, she recalled, remained 'a little more removed, nonetheless clearly caring of the community, but [he] never kind of dived in the same way we did'. He was, however, 'always very supportive' and 'learned to appreciate the fact that the skills that we brought to the situation enhanced his abilities'.[38]

Their immersion in Deaf culture, Boughman believed, was instrumental for gaining deaf people's trust in genetics, a science that in the past had often disapproved of their marriage or families, or had even tried to restrict them. Overcoming potential bias, she explained, was 'one of the reasons, especially, that Kathy Arnos and I opened ourselves up to the Deaf community'. They had to become 'part of the Deaf community' first, before they 'became geneticists to them'. For Boughman, this demonstrative humbleness and respect was not particular to working with deaf people, but rather a characteristic of 'human nature', a basic principle of cooperating with client communities: 'every time you demonstrate not only lack of bias, but acceptance and then move to clearly a respect, I think all of that ends up ... bringing you in'. It was important for her to signal that the scientist was not claiming a superior status, but required the community's help and knowledge.[39]

By the late 1970s then, Arnos, Boughman, and Nance had come to form a 'small supportive culture for each other', nourished and strengthen by the awareness of trying to accomplish something new that 'took some energy, took some effort'.[40] In the early 1980s, they realized several projects, including a long-term epidemiological study of students affected by Congenital Rubella Syndrome (CRS). During the 1970s and 1980s, children and teenagers with CRS formed a large and distinct group at schools for the deaf. Eighty-five per cent of students born in 1964/65 and enrolled in schools for the deaf were estimated to have CRS. Their specific health and education needs were still being explored. By the late 1970s, it had become clear that many of them experienced medical complications beyond the classical CRS triad of visual, auditory, and cardiac impairment. They also showed an unusually high rate of late-onset metabolic or endocrinological conditions, such as diabetes, thyroid dysfunction, or growth hormone deficiency. The reasons were unclear. Supported with an NIH grant from 1979 to 1984, Nance's team explored the link between CRS and diabetes, looking for potential genetic susceptibilities.[41]

Working with the rubella cohort brought the researchers into contact with the deaf communities around Gallaudet's Model Middle School and the Virginia and Maryland schools for the deaf; a contact they appreciated and explicitly sought. For Boughman and Arnos in particular visits to these schools were yet another opportunity to immerse themselves in Deaf culture and community. For Arnos, working with the rubella cohort reinforced her fascination with both the cultural and the biological sides of deafness and strengthened her conviction that only knowledge of both would lead to better services.

Similarly, for Boughman the experience of engaging with deaf students, of getting to know them as individuals, pointed to the necessity of direct communication and cultural sensitivity.[42]

Field trips in particular provided opportunities for immersion in Deaf culture and direct interaction with the community – for both Arnos and Boughman a crucial characteristic of a good geneticist. In dealing with students and their families, in entering the closed-off world of a residential school, their knowledge of ASL and ability to move between cultures were indispensable tools. Their ability to communicate in the students' language turned out to be an icebreaker, turning the outside scientists into more familiar figures. Students, Boughman emphasized, 'got to know us as people then, not just [as] the folks in the white coats' who 'drew their blood'.[43]

This approach removed the distance between scientist and object of research, the hierarchy between adult and teenager, and, not least, the difference between a hearing and a deaf person. It emphasized a cooperative model, in which both sides were needed for a successful study, and, eventually, better health care. Being able to communicate directly allowed her and Arnos to explain the purpose of the study to the teenage participants, to assuage fears about tests, to make sure that students really wanted to participate – and to offer them a way out if the prospect of needles and tests proved too uncomfortable. This was an important step beyond acquiring informed consent from parents. Such a cooperative model, Boughman believed, was not only ethically superior to a more paternalistic model of medical authority, but, by engaging in conversations with students and their families, also yielded a level of detail and textured information unattainable with only interpreters and questionnaires.[44]

To Arnos, field trips were among the project's most interesting and enjoyable features, to the point that she later remarked: 'I earned my PhD with field work!'[45] 'Field work' evokes images of ethnographers, anthropologists, and sociologists collecting folk tales or studying popular culture. In these disciplines, fieldwork has traditionally oscillated between immersion and identification with the study population on the one hand, and an analytical distance on the other. In genetics, too, there has been a long history of surveying rural, isolated areas, if not exotic locations, for inbreeding qualities and interesting traits. Historians have described how different types of data – family tales or family bibles, religious and family records, tissue or blood samples – became incorporated in genetic research, and how field work could create a research community of patients, families, and scientists. Such close cooperation tied scientists to the goals and values of a community, which could reach from searching for a cure to acknowledging that a trait might not require a cure after all.[46]

Arnos and Boughman's rubella fieldwork combined the ethnographic tradition of living among one's study population with the biomedical study of their traits. It resulted in a level of identification and assimilation that remained rare in biomedicine. Conducting field work among the Amish, famous Johns Hopkins geneticist Victor McKusick, for example, extracted different kinds of medical-genetic information, in exchange providing the Amish with better access to genetic diagnosis and services. McKusick, however, remained as much an outsider to the world and values of the Amish, as the Amish did to the world and values of medical genetics.[47] For Arnos and Boughman, on the other hand, their self-assigned role as intercultural ambassadors engendered a feeling of responsibility towards their client communities beyond medical or genetic needs. During their field trips to local schools for the deaf, they would spend time not only with children in the rubella cohort, but with students of all ages. For 'some of these [younger] kids', Boughman commented, 'we were the first hearing adults from the real world that knew sign language'. They 'were more than willing' to satisfy the children's curiosity about the strange phenomena of hearing adults who signed fluently, taking 'every ... chance to bridge the gap'.[48]

Although the study remained inconclusive on potential genetic susceptibility for rubella and diabetes, it emphasized the need for specialized health services for the rubella cohort – including genetics. A number of children and teenagers with CRS, the scientists realized, had actually been misdiagnosed. To a trained geneticist it was clear that they did not have rubella, but a genetic syndrome. This brought up difficult ethical considerations. What to tell them and their parents? How to provide them with a correct diagnosis and counsel them, without shaking their beliefs and identities, or raising guilt in their parents? The experience of coming across a group of genetically deaf teenagers who 'had not been identified, not been counseled', reinforced Arnos' belief in 'the need for setting up services within the deaf community', which provided 'sensitive information-giving and sensitive counseling'.[49] She, Nance, and Boughman had steadily pursued this goal in the previous years. There were, however, still obstacles to making available such services to deaf individuals. The lack of ASL signs for genetic terminology was one of them.

By the 1980s, geneticists had probed deaf people's pedigrees, medical, family, or school records for about a century. They had taken audiograms, ordered medical examinations, and advised deaf individuals and their families on suitable reproductive behaviour. Yet – and this was telling for the on-going lack of communication and exchange between researchers and deaf objects of research – they had not bothered to translate genetic concepts into the native language of their research population. If geneticists or medical staff used sign language interpreters, or, more rarely, signed themselves, genetic terminology usually was fingerspelled.

In American Sign Language, fingerspelling – spelling each letter in the manual alphabet rather than using a single or compound sign – is used for proper names, places, or titles, and more generally for rarely used terms. Most of these acquire specific signs as needed. Many science-specific terms fall into this category. This was even truer in a period before a sizable number of deaf people had entered medicine and biomedical research, and when basic science education at schools for the deaf was chronically lacking. This lack made signed conversations about genetics cumbersome, especially for non-native signers like Boughman and Arnos. They lamented in 1983 that 'communicating in a language, in which all specialized terms must be spelled out because specific signs for these terms do not exist can be unproductive and frustrating'.[50]

Collaborating with a team of Gallaudet linguists and the DC area Deaf community, Boughman and Arnos set out to develop 'acceptable manual signs for genetic terminology' to fill this gap.[51] They first gave talks on genetics and genetic counselling to different groups, including native deaf signers, registered interpreters, and hearing people with diverse levels of signing ability. They surveyed the audience for which genetic terms already existed or were considered necessary. For some concepts, they found existing terms, including a sign for Usher syndrome. Signs for other genetic syndromes were then based on the same concept. Usher syndrome was signed with the right hand in a U shape at the level of the forehead, then forming an S shape at the chin level; Down syndrome repeated this pattern with a D and an S shape. From these terms and suggestions, the project team assembled a preliminary set of twenty-three signs. A group of Gallaudet linguists and students from science and linguistic classes then evaluated a videotape of each sign for its 'conceptualization, ease of formation, clarity, and necessity'. In the end, twelve signs remained. These were published in the 1983 booklet *Signs for Genetic Counseling*.[52] For each term there was a photo of the sign, signing instructions, and a definition. The booklet thus not only was a dictionary, but also an introduction to the most important concepts of genetics. Signs included different syndromes – Usher, Waardenburg, and Down syndrome as 'the most common chromosomal problem seen in newborns' – as well as genetic terminology such as chromosome, dominant, or recessive, and the increasingly common diagnostic technology of amniocentesis.[53]

The booklet also introduced the sign for genetics, defining it as 'the scientific study of heredity; the study of traits in the family'.[54] Notably, this was a neutral definition, one that aimed at the study of genetic traits rather than the prevention of a single trait, such as deafness. Incorporating genetic terms into the native language of the target community signalled a new dimension of bringing genetic knowledge to deaf people. Developing ASL signs for genetic concepts meant adapting genetics to Deaf culture; but reversely it also meant popularizing these concepts to the Deaf community. In this spirit, the booklet noted that a growing awareness of genetics would increase deaf people's need for genetic counselling and help determine 'the chances' – note the neutralized terminology – of having deaf or hearing children.[55]

The project mirrored Boughman's and Arnos' belief in the equality of ASL as a language not only capable of expressing abstract concepts, but best suited to do so when signing deaf people were concerned. Relying on native signers' linguistic expertise, it equalized, or even reversed the relationship between geneticists and their target population. Boughman believed that signalling their reliance on Deaf native speakers helped the project gain respect from the Deaf community: 'it was part of being accepted, the fact that here were these scientists that understood that there was more to it than just their science content, that we wanted to move forward, we wanted to do it right, we wanted to do it their way'. Describing the project as a mutual learning process, she later called it '[o]ne of the best things that I ever did in my career'.[56] The cooperation with linguists gave her new insights, and collaborating to find new terms created a sense of accomplishment, an emotional process of identification with, and participation in, Deaf culture and community.

Taking genetics to the heart of American Deaf culture: the Gallaudet Genetic Services Center

By the early 1980s, Nance, Boughman, and Arnos had pursued the goal of making their science accessible and acceptable to deaf people for several years. Arnos and Boughman in particular had acted as ambassadors between the medical-genetic and the deaf communities. Despite these efforts, however, they still found the relationship between the two groups unsatisfactory. 'Nobody knew sign language', Boughman said of her hearing colleagues. 'Nobody crossed into Deaf culture. The deaf didn't come into our clinics', just as geneticists were not 'going into the Deaf community and offering their services'. Other geneticists 'just weren't in there'. The 'language' and 'cultural barrier' caused 'assumptions' that were 'made on both sides'. On the side of geneticists, she felt, there were 'paternalistic assumptions' that deaf people 'don't want to know' about genetics. On 'the inside', from deaf people, she detected 'the fear' that 'they're going to tell us we're bad people'.[57] With the

Gallaudet Genetic Services Center, established in 1984, they hoped to close this cultural and linguistic gap.

Finishing her PhD in 1983, Arnos followed the rubella cohort from school to Gallaudet, where she served as research coordinator and liaison between the Medical College of Virginia, where Nance now headed the genetics department, and the Gallaudet Research Institute. She soon took part in other campus activities that gave her an opportunity to teach and counsel. Working in the DC area, she also came into contact with the DC Genetic Services Program, a regional consortium of four genetics centres. Supported by the Department of Human Services (DHS), it aimed to bring genetic services – testing, counselling, and education – to disadvantaged groups. Its programme for Special Projects of Regional and National Significance (SPRANS) solicited proposals addressing 'linguistic and cultural barriers to genetic counseling'.[58] Deaf people, Arnos believed, clearly fell into this category. She submitted a proposal for SPRANS funding for 'an Innovative Approach to Genetic Counseling Services for the Deaf'.[59]

Portraying deaf people as a group in need of specialized genetic services, the proposal showed the appeal of a sociocultural minority model, yet also its limitations when it came to legitimizing genetic services. The proposal defined deafness as 'a debilitating disorder that poses cultural and language barriers that severely limit access to genetics services'. The limiting – indeed, the disabling – effects of deafness thus were both physical and sociological: Physically, deafness was a 'debilitating disorder', the 'most common physical impairment in the Unites States today', with 2,000–4,000 deaf infants born per year, and an estimated total of 1.6 million 'affected individuals'. Sociologically, deaf people were an 'articulate minority in our society'. Yet this status, too, was tied to physical characteristics. Unlike 'other U.S. minorities whose linguistic isolation is based solely on the use of a foreign language', deaf people's status as a minority depended on a physical and potentially genetic trait.[60] While many deaf people did not consider deafness itself pathological, other, associated traits were considered pathological by both geneticists and most deaf people. Usher syndrome or Jervell and Lange-Nielsen syndrome (a potentially fatal heart condition), for example, Arnos argued, demonstrated the need for timely diagnosis and adequate medical, educational, and rehabilitation services.[61]

It was thus their genetic make-up that made deaf people a 'genetic high-risk group' – yet it was society, Arnos wrote, that had created 'cultural and language barriers' to genetic services. Genetics professionals in particular had failed to learn about Deaf culture and failed to push for accessible genetic services. As she wrote: 'The failure to provide needed diagnostic and counseling services at a time when millions are spent to screen for genetic diseases that have an incidence of less than 1 in 10.000 in the population ... is a national shame that bears mute testimony to the political impotence of the deaf.'[62] This was familiar fund-raising rhetoric in the history of disease awareness campaigns in general, and the push for genetic deafness research in particular. Appealing to a sense of neglect and misguided effort, it created a sense of urgency, singling out deafness and deaf people as particularly worthy of attention.

The proposal was successful. In 1984, the Genetic Services Center began operating as part of the Gallaudet's student health services. Arnos headed the centre, supported by a secretary and a part-time clinical nurse fluent in sign language. Over the years and with extended funding, staff grew to include more genetic counsellors. Beyond this core staff, the centre was supported by external partners, including Walter Nance and Joann Boughman (now at the University of Maryland).[63] Cooperation with the DC Genetic Services Program helped maximize resources and extended the centre's reach beyond the immediate campus community. Education, screening, counselling, and research circumscribed its scope. Screening served the double purpose of providing genetic counselling and of collecting data to add to Nance's genetic deafness database at MCV.[64]

An important first step in culturally sensitive, non-directive counselling was to make sure that counsellor and client could understand each other. Thus, when an individual or couple came to the centre, establishing communication preferences was a crucial first step. The vast majority of clients preferred ASL, yet the centre also provided other options, including lip-reading or signed English. Providing 'culturally neutral terminology',[65] rather than describing deafness as a risk or pathological state, was another important point. Similarly, it was important to learn why a client was seeking genetic evaluation in first place. There was a wide range of motivations, from medical or reproductive concerns to plain curiosity. Some clients wanted to learn their chances for hearing or deaf children, some explicitly wished for one or the other, some simply wanted to know why they were deaf.[66] In fact, Arnos noted in 1992, the majority of clients 'had sought counseling because of curiosity', and stated that 'their reproductive decisions would not be altered' by genetic information.[67] In encouraging this curiosity, staff actively built and fed into a sense of genetics as part of a deaf person's identity, of one's self to be discovered. Medical considerations were more pronounced in clients with syndromic deafness, who were concerned about passing on their condition to their children. Clients also sought genetic counselling for conditions unrelated to deafness, such as Tay Sachs disease, cancer risk, or rare genetic conditions.[68]

There was, Boughman recalled, 'a hunger for knowledge of why and how' a person was deaf. Interest was so great, that 'we learned very quickly that ... we weren't going to have to sell this to anybody ... they were lining up to come see us'. Many of the first clients were not students, but faculty members curious about the new addition to campus. Once the first clients had been seen and left with a good impression, 'word travel[ed] fast'. Visiting the centre, Boughman observed, became an 'acceptable activity to do', something people would do to satisfy their curiosity about this new institution and its services without having 'to be at all surreptitious'.[69] Indeed, of the 659 clients who sought genetic evaluation and counselling from October 1984 to December 1990, most were self-referred. The majority of them were students and young couples, with a mean age of twenty-three years.[70]

Once staff had established why a client sought counselling and how they preferred to communicate, they gathered relevant information such as family histories and audiograms, and conducted physical examinations. Ideally, this resulted in a definite diagnosis. Yet in about one in four cases, the type of deafness could not be identified. By the mid-1980s, more than 100 forms of genetic deafness had been identified; by the early 1990s, the number had grown to about 200. At the same time, however, many other forms remained un- or under-defined. Diagnosis was particularly difficult if the client was the only deaf person in the family. Families with many deaf individuals also were a challenge. The centre, Arnos recalled, would see 'a lot of big deaf families ... where everyone was deaf and initially, it could have been dominant, it could have been recessive – we couldn't figure it out'.[71] In such cases, generalized empirical risk tables provided the closest assessment. Nance and his students Susan Pilant Rose and Frederick R. Bieber had produced such tables for deafness. They provided the likelihood for certain outcomes, based on a large body of statistic data – more than 49,000 children born to more than 12,000 families. If, for example, a deaf child was born to hearing parents, deafness could have genetic or environmental causes, and the initial likelihood of having another deaf child was estimated as 25 per cent. If another deaf or hearing children was born to the family, the statistical likelihood increased or lowered accordingly.[72]

The inability to provide a definite diagnosis might well have been seen as a failure. After all, most clients came to the centre to learn about the cause of their deafness. Yet it also reinforced the notion of genetic counselling as an intense encounter between counsellor and clients, which had as many emotional as medical benefits. Counselling, Arnos suggested, evoking well-established themes, was as much psychotherapy as fact-giving. 'Many benefits of genetic counseling', she and her co-workers echoed Nance or Kallmann almost verbatim, 'are unrelated to reproductive decisions'. For hearing parents, counselling could 'help to relieve the guilt that some hearing parents may have carried around with them for many years'. It could also 'help the family to accept and adjust to the birth of a deaf child'. Conversely, in deaf parents, it could 'help them to deal with any fears they may have about raising a hearing child'.[73] Genetic counselling, then, was to be a service that took seriously, and sought to alleviate, clients' fears, questions, and concerns.

Retreating from decisive, directive, or definite positions, genetic counselling instead gained authority as a helping and supportive profession. In doing so, it claimed a mediator position, a point of first contact for parents learning about deafness, meeting their need for support and information with referrals to educational and psychological resources. Genetic counselling, Arnos and her co-workers cautioned, 'emphasizes informed decision making and provision of medical, psychological, and social support; genetic counseling is not advice giving'. Successful counselling required the counsellor 'to be aware of the context in which counseling is given and respect cultural and linguistic differences of the patient'. Just as in psychotherapy, it required that the professional engaged in a critical self-reflection of his or her own values and emotions during the counselling process. Consequently, deaf clients' preference for deaf or hearing children was not to be seen as deviant. Rather it had become a testing case for the much-discussed dogma of late twentieth-century genetic counselling: non-directiveness.[74]

Marketing their services directly to deaf people and their families, and operating in an increasingly politicized environment of Deaf activism on and off campus, the centre, too, was more explicitly political. It claimed an empowering dimension to genetic self-knowledge. Two brochures from the 1980s and early 1990s drew a direct line from acquiring individual genetic knowledge to self-determination and empowerment. 'Do you wonder about ... the cause of your hearing loss? The chance that you might have a hearing impaired child?' one of them asked, and offered the centre's services.

With its purposefully neutral terminology – chance instead of risk, wonder instead of worry, acquiring knowledge instead of prevention – the brochure cast learning about one's genetics as a positive step, something one might do out of curiosity rather than medical necessity. While genetic evaluation might provide a definite diagnosis, its implications – 'the impact it may have on you and your family in the future' – were left open, conditional upon individual beliefs and circumstances.[75] Yet it also acquired an explicitly political dimension: To 'become informed' was to 'become empowered', another brochure asserted, and explained that 'this is your opportunity to learn more about emerging issues in genetics and learn more about yourself'. And it continued ominously: 'advances in genetics will no doubt impact Deaf culture'. The implied call for action was clear: if genetics would impact Deaf culture, it was

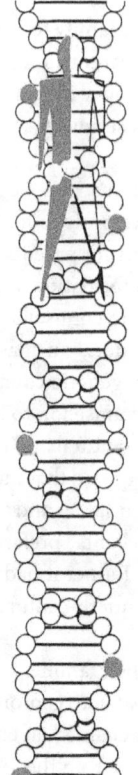

As a hearing impaired person, have you ever wondered about:

O The cause of your hearing impairment?

O The chances that you might have hearing impaired children?

As a hearing person, have you asked about:

● Why some children are born with a hearing loss?

● What caused a hearing loss in a member of your family?

● Whether you might have hearing impaired children?

These and other questions can be answered by genetic services, which are available to you and your family. These services include:

O Medical evaluation to find the causes of hearing impairment

O Genetic counseling

O Support services

Figure 5 'Have you ever wondered?', detail from a Gallaudet Genetic Services Center Brochure, c. mid-1990s (reprinted with kind permission of Gallaudet University University Archives)

imperative for deaf individuals to become informed in order to assert their genetic and cultural identity in society.[76]

Conclusion

In many ways, genetic counselling for deafness at Gallaudet looked very different from what Walter Nance had practised at the Wilkerson Center in the late 1960s. At the same time, it built upon long-standing themes and developments in the history of genetic deafness research: the notion that deaf people were under-served and under-informed about genetics; and that learning

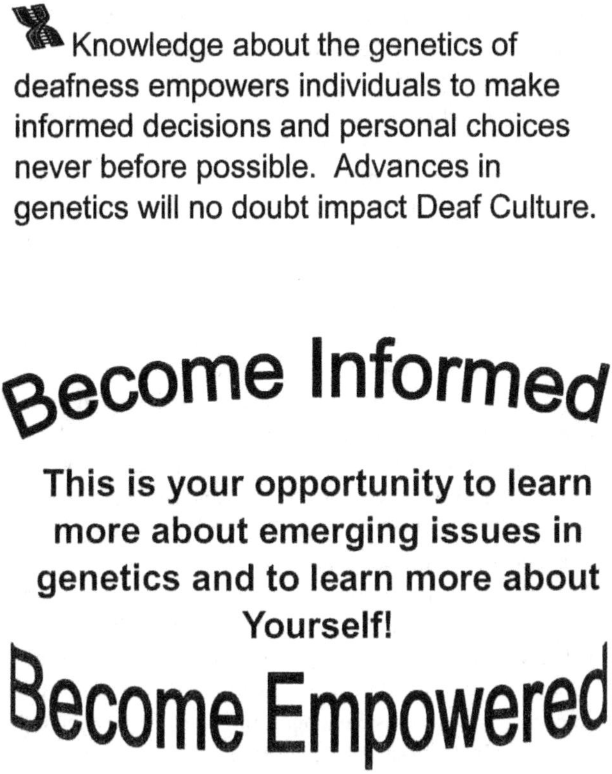

> Knowledge about the genetics of deafness empowers individuals to make informed decisions and personal choices never before possible. Advances in genetics will no doubt impact Deaf Culture.

Become Informed

This is your opportunity to learn more about emerging issues in genetics and to learn more about Yourself!

Become Empowered

Figure 6 'Become empowered', detail from a Gallaudet Genetic Services Center Brochure, c. mid-1990s (reprinted with kind permission of Gallaudet University University Archives)

about their genetic make-up would benefit their lives and futures. What had changed significantly, however, where assumptions about the nature of these benefits, and about who was at fault for their supposed state of genetic under-information. Now, geneticists claimed that it was their colleagues who had neglected to take into account the special needs and sensitivities of deaf people.

In their claims about neglect and about the empowering dimension of genetic knowledge geneticists mobilized the long-standing motive of a progression from ignorance to knowledge. Since the late nineteenth century, professionals had tried to instil in deaf people an awareness of their hereditary make-up, generally with the goal of prevention and normalization. Yet in genetics, what was to be prevented and how so became a matter of discussion. Non-directive, psychosocial genetic counselling meant that, at least in theory, it was the client who decided which services to use, which decisions to make – and what was a pathological condition in the first place. Nance had early on promoted the emotional benefits of counselling. Like other geneticists in the 1960s and 1970s, he advocated genetics as an instrument to counter the blame and stigma of disability, and to 'complete' the family with a 'normal' child. His deaf clients, however, questioned what a 'normal' family or child was in first place. Such an encounter did not necessarily lead to a mental reorientation. But by the 1970s, researchers, who, like Nance, were curious and wanted to learn more, had an advantage over their colleagues even a decade earlier: there was now a growing, easily available body of research on Deaf people as a sociolinguistic-cultural minority. Just as important, Deaf activists and artists had become more visible in public, claiming their right to sign language and Deaf culture. Both of these developments culminated at Gallaudet. Indeed, the campus had become a locus of research that attracted scientists from beyond the traditional field of deaf education, and provided opportunities for first-hand experiences with Deaf culture.

Together with a reorientation in genetic counselling towards client-centredness, this visibility and availability of Deaf culture facilitated an approach that valued deaf people's perspectives. It was necessary, Nance, Boughman, and Arnos thought, to assimilate themselves and their science to the deaf community, purposefully obscuring the line between experts and objects of research. In doing so, they reversed established notions of blame and resistance. Geneticists had anxiously watched deaf people's reproductive patterns, chastising them for 'irresponsible' marriages and ignorance of hereditary principles. This was wrong, Nance, Arnos, and Boughman believed. It was not that deaf people were disinterested in genetics, or even were resisting learning about it. Rather, it was genetics professionals who had failed to provide them with meaningful services and communication, and had resisted learning about Deaf culture. It was professional ignorance that had turned deaf people into a neglected population in first place. Conveying a sense of atonement for past mistakes and misconceptions, this self-portrayal put geneticists in a strategic mediator position. To the deaf community, it signalled remorseful willingness to overcome past biases. To genetic professionals it offered a way to improve their services, which resonated with contemporary ideals of community health care, patient autonomy, and informed decision-making.

Turning (potential) patients into clients and consumers, the Genetic Services Centre portrayed genetics as a service customized to the beliefs of a minority that was often still at odds with majority perceptions of deafness.

This set them apart from other patient–expert communities and alliances that formed during the time, which often rallied around the search for a cure or biomedical solutions. The Genetic Services Center, on the other hand, no longer aimed at a specific outcome – the prevention of deafness – but rather identified deafness as a one of many possible cultural and genetic states. It was genetic informed-ness and self-awareness that mattered – no longer (necessarily) what one did with it. Nevertheless, underlying this primacy of information over action, there was the assumption that acquiring genetic self-awareness would change one's behaviour, if only to turn an unaware individual into an informed consumer of genetic services. This had important implications. Being informed about one's genetic self was not only a form of controlling individual fate, of finding an important part of oneself, but became part of political empowerment, too. The informed consumer of genetic services could become an advocate representing the values of a sociocultural minority.

Whereas the eugenicists of the first part of the century legitimized their research as an improvement of race and humankind, geneticists now portrayed their work as a matter of empowering individuals and of ending minority discrimination, and themselves as activists for a more just, accessible health care for neglected, underserved populations. Casting geneticists in the ambivalent, multi-layered role of a scientist-advocate, this gave a new spin to the notion of genetic counselling as a helping science. Supporting their clients' identities, even if they diverged from majority culture, genetics became a supportive science of late twentieth-century identity politics.

Notes

1 W. E. Nance, 'Genetic counseling of hereditary deafness: an unmet need', in Bess (ed.), *Childhood Deafness*, pp. 211–16, here p. 212.
2 W. E. Nance, 'Genetic counseling for the hearing impaired', *Audiology: Official Organ of the International Society of Audiology*, 10:4 (1971), 222–33, here 222.
3 W. E. Nance, 'The principles and practice of genetic counseling', *The Annals of Otology, Rhinology, and Laryngology*, 80:2 (1971), 246–54, here 250.
4 *Ibid.*
5 'Oral history interview with Walter Nance', 11 September 2006, Sewanee, TN. Interviewer: Nathaniel Comfort. UCLA-Johns Hopkins Oral History of Human Genetics Project, pp. 1–3, 9.
6 *Ibid.*, pp. 28–9.
7 *Ibid.*, pp. 3, 29, 30, 32.
8 *Ibid.*, pp. 3–4, 58.
9 *Ibid.*, pp. 1, 3–5, 37–8, 66–8.

10 F. McConnell, *The Bill Wilkerson Hearing and Speech Center, its Origin and its Development* (Nashville, TN: The Center, 1978), pp. 78, 87.
11 Ibid., pp. 69, 115–18. Also see the papers of the centre's medical social worker Anne J. Sweeney, Eskind Biomedical Library Special Collections, Vanderbilt University Medical Center, Nashville, TN, Anne J. Sweeney Papers, in particular, F. McConnell, A. Sweeney, A. C. McLeod, M. E. Glasscock, P. H. Ward, W. E. Nance, and J. Cherrie, *Experimental Studies in Hereditary Deafness. Final Report. Grant No. R01 06408*. January 1975. US Department of Health, Education, and Welfare. National Institute of Neurological Diseases and Stroke.
12 'Oral history interview with Walter Nance', pp. 36–7.
13 For the more recent history of Gallaudet, see D. F. Armstrong, *The History of Gallaudet University: 150 years of a Deaf American Institution* (Washington DC: Gallaudet University Press, 2014), pp. 71–103.
14 'Oral history interview with Walter Nance', pp. 2, 3.
15 Armstrong, *History of Gallaudet*, pp. 72–5.
16 See Gallaudet University Archives, Departmental Files, Folder 35, File 72.1, 'Office of Demographic Studies reports 1977 (No.1)'. For the history and purpose of the annual survey see M. Marschark and P. E. Spencer (eds), *Oxford Handbook of Deaf Studies, Language, and Education* (Oxford: Oxford University Press, 2003), p. 22.
17 Schein, *The Deaf Community*, pp. 3, 94. For Schein's work and advocacy, see Anon., 'Obituaries. Jerome D. Schein', *The Hearing Journal*, 63:6 (June 2010), 56.
18 Nance et al., 'Opportunities for genetic counseling', 330–1.
19 W. E. Nance, 'Studies of hereditary deafness', *Volta Review*, 78 (1976), 6–11, here 9.
20 For these developments see C. Padden and T. Humphries, *Inside Deaf Culture* (Cambridge, MA: Harvard University Press, 2005), pp. 79–99; Gannon et al., *Deaf Heritage*, pp. 377–93.
21 'Oral history interview with Joann Boughman', Adelphi, MD, 27 August 2013. Interviewer: Marion Schmidt. J. A. Boughman, 'Population genetic studies of retinitis pigmentosa' (PhD dissertation, Indiana University, 1978).
22 Stern, *Telling Genes*, pp. 15, 24, 102–22.
23 'Oral history interview with Joann Boughman'.
24 Ibid.
25 Ibid.
26 Ibid.
27 Ibid.
28 For the growing popularity of ASL among hearing people and the media presence of deaf artists see Gannon et al., *Deaf Heritage*, pp. 345–56, 372–6; Baynton, *Forbidden Signs*, pp. 154–7; Padden and Humphries, *Inside Deaf Culture*, 109–19, 157–63.
29 'Oral history interview with Joann Boughman'.
30 For risk in genetic counselling see Stern, *Telling Genes*, pp. 37–8.

31 'Oral history interview with Joann Boughman'.
32 *Ibid.*
33 *Ibid.*
34 *Ibid.*
35 S. Lyons, 'College program leads way in deaf education. Western Maryland offers first Master's in sign language', *Baltimore Sun* (4 May 1998); R. J. Anderson, C. E. Keller, and J. M. Karp, *Enhancing Diversity. Educators with Disabilities* (Washington, DC: Gallaudet University Press, 1998), pp. 242–6.
36 'Oral history interview with Kathleen Shaver Arnos', Washington, DC, 9 October 2012. Interviewer: Marion Schmidt.
37 *Ibid.*
38 'Oral history interview with Joann Boughman'.
39 *Ibid.*
40 *Ibid.*
41 See e.g. K. A. Shaver, J. A. Boughman, and W. E. Nance, 'LA Antigens in the congenital Rubella syndrome', *Disease Markers*, 2 (1984), 381–91; K. A. Shaver, J. A. Boughman, and W. E. Nance, 'Congenital rubella syndrome and diabetes: a review of epidemiologic, genetic, and immunologic factors', *American Annals of the Deaf*, 130:6 (1985), 526–32.
42 'Oral history interview with Kathleen Shaver Arnos'; 'Oral history interview with Joann Boughman'.
43 'Oral history interview with Joann Boughman'.
44 *Ibid.*
45 'Oral history interview with Kathleen Shaver Arnos'.
46 Historians have described such fieldwork in various communities, see e.g. Lindee, 'Genetic disease'; Lindee, *Moments of Truth*, pp. 59–88; Wexler, *Mapping Fate*.
47 For McKusick see Lindee, *Moments of Truth*, pp. 62, 77.
48 'Oral history interview with Joann Boughman'.
49 'Oral history interview with Kathleen Shaver Arnos'.
50 J. A. Boughman and K A. Shaver, 'Responsibilities in genetic counseling for the deaf', *American Journal of Human Genetics*, 35:6 (1983), 1317–19, here 1317.
51 *Ibid.*
52 See Gallaudet College, *Signs for Genetic Counseling: For Genetic Counselors, Clients, and Sign Language Interpreters* (Washington, DC: National Academy of Gallaudet College, 1983).
53 *Ibid.*, p. 4.
54 *Ibid.*
55 *Ibid.*, p. 1.
56 'Oral history interview with Joann Boughman'.
57 *Ibid.*
58 'Oral history interview with Kathleen Shaver Arnos'.
59 Division of Research, Gallaudet College, 'Proposal: Demonstration of an

Innovative Approach to Genetic Counseling Services for the Deaf Population to Department of Health and Human Services Bureau of Health Care Delivery and Assistance Division of Maternal and Child Health 5600 Fishers Lange Rockville, Maryland 20857 by Division of Research, Gallaudet College' (Gallaudet College, Washington, DC: Division of Research, May 1 1984).
60 Ibid., pp. 2–3.
61 Ibid., pp. 2, 6–7.
62 Ibid., pp. 3, 7.
63 Ibid., pp. 17–8. Also see 'Oral history interview with Kathleen Shaver Arnos'.
64 'Oral history interview with Kathleen Shaver Arnos'.
65 Arnos et al., 'Innovative approach', 345. In 1992, 90 per cent of clients preferred to communicate in ASL.
66 'Oral history interview with Kathleen Shaver Arnos'.
67 Arnos et al., 'Innovative approach', 349.
68 'Oral history interview with Kathleen Shaver Arnos'. Also see K. S. Arnos, 'The implications of genetic testing for deafness', *Ear and Hearing*, 24:4 (2003), 324–31, here 325.
69 'Oral history interview with Joann Boughman'.
70 Arnos et al., 'Innovative approach', 347–9.
71 'Oral history interview with Kathleen Shaver Arnos'; Arnos et al., 'Innovative approach', 347; K. S. Arnos, J. Israel, and M. Cunningham, 'Genetic counseling of the deaf', *Annals of the New York Academy of Sciences*, 630 (1991), 212–22, here 215.
72 See F. R. Bieber and W. E. Nance, 'Hereditary hearing loss', in L. G. Jackson and R. N. Schimke (eds), *Clinical Genetics: A Source Book for Physicians* (New York: Wiley, 1979), pp. 443–61, here 456–8. Also see the theses of Rose and Bieber: S. P. Rose, 'Genetic studies of profound prelingual deafness' (PhD dissertation, Indiana University, 1975); F. R. Bieber, 'Genetic studies of questionnaire data from a residential school for the deaf' (PhD dissertation, Virginia Commonwealth University, 1981). For risk evaluation in cases where the cause of deafness could not be identified also see G. R. Fraser, *The Causes of Profound Deafness in Childhood: A Study of 3,535 Individuals with Severe Hearing Loss Present at Birth or of Childhood Onset* (Baltimore, MD: Johns Hopkins University Press, 1976), pp. 336–42.
73 Arnos et al., 'Genetic counseling', 215.
74 Ibid.; Arnos et al., 'Innovative approach', 345.
75 Gallaudet University Archives, Departmental Files, Box 28, Folder 99.1, 'Genetic Services Center, Brochures', n. d. The brochure was printed before the change of name and status from Gallaudet College to Gallaudet University in 1986.
76 Ibid. This second brochure was printed after Gallaudet became a university, c. late 1980s or early 1990s. The argument for the empowering dimension of genetic knowledge is made more explicitly in the later work of Arnos, Boughman, and Nance. See e.g. W. E. Nance, 'The epidemiology of hereditary deafness: the impact of connexin 26 on the size and structure of the deaf community', in J. V. Van Cleve

(ed.), *Genetics, Disability and Deafness* (Washington DC: Gallaudet University Press, 2004), pp. 94–105; K. S. Arnos, 'Attitudes of deaf individuals towards genetic testing', *American Journal of Medical Genetics*, 130:17 (2004), 17–21, here 19.

CONCLUSION: FROM BELL TO BIODIVERSITY

In 2003, Walter Nance contemplated the future of the American Deaf community. Referring to the 'social and ethical aspects of genetic deafness', he speculated that with recent advances in biomedicine, 'Deaf culture may well disappear in our country by the end of this century'. Yet, he argued, it was not genetics that Deaf people had to fear most. Rather it was cochlear implant technology that 'almost certainly represents a much greater threat to deaf culture than genetic testing'.[1] This was a statement revealing of geneticists' changing self-perception.

Since cochlear implants (CIs) entered the health care market in the mid-1980s, and especially since the 1990s, when they were approved for infants and toddlers, they have been seen as a kind of (instant) cure for neurosensoral deafness. They have also intensified old divisions. Once more, deaf children are in the middle of a highly emotional debate about their identity, belonging, and future, about whether deafness is something to be fixed or cherished. For CI professionals – neurosurgeons, audiologists, or speech therapists – they spell out a future in which the child is made quasi-hearing via technology and hard therapeutic work. And thus, once more, sign languages have been declared obsolete, no longer needed except for those children not suitable for or succeeding with a CI. Unsurprisingly, these claims have made CIs controversial in the Deaf community. Deaf activists have charged parents of making their child undergo risky and unnecessary surgery, of oppressing Deaf identities, and making it into something it is not.[2] With a generation of children and teenagers now growing up with CIs, the long-term impact on Deaf culture and identity remains to be seen. Yet when geneticists such as Nance make claims about the relative danger of cochlear implants versus genetics, they create a simplified scenario of competing technological threats, which is more telling of their self-portrayal than analytical about the social impact of technology.

It is also, perhaps, wishful thinking. Despite a greater awareness of Deaf identities, science and society at large still view deaf people's reproductive life with suspicion. In 2002, for example, the American couple Sharon Duchesneau and Candace McCullough became the probably most publicized and controversial instance of two deaf people wanting to expand their family. The couple's first child was deaf, and although they would have welcomed a child of any hearing status, this was an outcome they hoped for their second child, too. To improve their odds, they first contacted a sperm bank, yet were told that deaf men were not eligible donors. They then approached a male friend from a multi-generational deaf family, who had a form of dominant genetic deafness. When their son was born, he indeed turned out to be deaf – a cause of joy for the Duchesneau-McCullough family... and of intense public debate over disability, reproductive rights, and parental responsibility. Reactions were highly emotional and ranged from accusations of creating designer babies to charges of selfishness and child abuse. Although public attention on the Duchesneau-McCullough family has faded, they have become a popular – and oddly disembodied – teaching case in bioethics, disability, and Deaf studies.[3]

In the early twenty-first century, then, the old debates over how and what deaf people should be, and what kind of children they should have, are far from being resolved. They continue around the meaning of disability, disease, and suffering, citizenship and identity, scientific authority and intervention. However, unlike in the first half of the twentieth century, sympathies and alliance are no longer clearly drawn between deaf people on the one side, and hearing professionals and society on the other. In recent decades, Deaf culture and community have found a place in a more multi-cultural, diverse America – certainly controversial or offensive to some, but not necessarily more or less so than other minority cultures and identities. And unlike hearing professionals in earlier decades, those interested in sociocultural models of deafness and disability now have available for their (re)orientation a myriad of books and websites, signing deaf individuals in media and art, the fields of Deaf and disability studies, and, not least, a greater number of deaf colleagues in all kinds of professions.

This book explained why some American geneticists came to identify with a sociocultural model of deafness, and in turn, also why some other fields still mostly pursue a pathological-curative worldview. This situation is the result of the developments traced here, moving in an apparent paradox: as knowledge about (hereditary) deafness expanded, so did opinions on what to do about it. Over time, different ideas about deafness could align with different beliefs about what heredity research meant and should achieve. These changing alliances between different disciplines profoundly influenced how genetic knowledge was read and applied. Genetic deafness researchers collaborated or came in contact with professionals in numerous other fields, who, over the course of the twentieth century, claimed expertise of deafness and deaf people: physicians, otologists, and audiologists, teachers, sociologists, and linguists, philosophers, psychologists, and psychiatrists, rehabilitation workers, and counsellors.

Institutional context was crucial, as I have shown by example of oralist schools, psychiatric institutions, hearing-and-speech centres, and of Gallaudet as a centre of Deaf culture, activism, and research. How deafness and deaf people were seen in these contexts varied immensely, from the close and paternalistic long-term relationship between teachers and students, to considering deaf people as an interesting but mostly anonymous research population, to partners in improving health care services for a minority. More so than with other research populations, communication – or lack thereof – was a key issue, enmeshed in hardened ideological battles about the nature of thought, language, and humanness.

The history of deafness during the first two thirds of the twentieth century has often been written as one of unquestioned and uniform medicalization and pathologization. Yet underneath this apparently monolithic surface, different approaches and perceptions of deafness and deaf people formed, preceding and preparing later shifts and divisions. It is important to understand these approaches in their historical context, in all their complexities and ambivalence. It is also important to keep in mind the gap between claims to scientific progress and reality. Throughout the century and into the present, claims about the prognostic, diagnostic, and therapeutic powers of genetics have far outreached reality – yet the fact that these claims were appealing speak to the larger appeal of scientific solutions when it comes to funding, to public or academic support.

As a leading oralist institution, the Clarke School provides a good example of these complexities. Its self-portrayal as an institution incorporating cutting-edge science was essential to its story of helping deaf children succeed as quasi-hearing. This was a story also appealing to the outside researchers with whom Clarke collaborated since the establishment of its research department in 1928. Yet they also brought in their own assumptions about deafness, and their research often pursued goals quite different from the school's oralist assimilation. Mainly interested in social dynamics and interpersonal relationships, psychologists Fritz and Grace Moore Heider came to define deaf people as a sociological and phenomenological minority already in the 1940s. Concluding that deaf people should not be measured by hearing standards, their research ironically undermined basic oralist beliefs. Although ignored by the school, the Heiders' work provided an important precedent for the social minority model of deafness developing in the 1950s and 1960s.

Eugenicists and geneticists shared the school's concerns about hereditary deafness – yet did not necessarily agree what to do about it. Madge Macklin's public-health approach to eradicating pathological traits – if necessary by restricting the rights of carriers – was worlds removed from the school's holistic vision of heredity counselling as yet another means of integrating deaf students into hearing society by eradicating, as much as possible, their difference. Nevertheless, despite these differences oralist educators formed an alliance with eugenics and early medical genetics over the apparent truism that it was best for deaf people not to marry each other.

By the 1960s, however, this alliance weakened, ironically because the 1950s and 1960s were a watershed moment in understanding genetic deafness. Applying the latest research from cytogenetics, biochemistry, or biomedical computing, researchers began to tease out more generalizable patterns from their generation-spanning collection of pedigrees. They identified an ever-growing number of syndromes and speculated about the number of genes involved in hearing loss. Although individual diagnosis remained difficult, if not impossible, geneticists felt increasingly confident to predict that two deaf people were unlikely to have the same kind of deafness, and thus would not pass it on. Consequently, from a geneticist's point of view, there was no reason to advise them against having children, much less against marriage. In the larger refashioning of post-World War II genetics as a democratic science, this was an instance where genetic counselling could help foster 'normal' family life. For the oralist educator, on the other hand, deaf intermarriage still meant a failure to assimilate to the hearing world.

The mid-century decades were also pivotal in developing more relational and psychosocial approaches to deafness and disability. They were, to some degree, attractive to geneticists, who, with the advent of non-directive counselling, looked for insights to understanding clients' emotions and responses. Of course, taking a more psychosocial approach did not necessarily mean giving up older eugenic goals and rhetoric. It facilitated more client-centred definitions of normalcy and pathology, but also revealed geneticists' lingering anxiety over leaving reproductive decisions to patients. It also meant a shift in goals: with the rise of non-directive counselling, geneticists no longer necessarily aimed at preventing a certain condition. Rather they advocated achieving genetic awareness – and assumed that, from there on, clients would come to a 'rational' decision on their own. Such genetic awareness, geneticists claimed, was essential for the modern citizen, and something to which everyone was entitled – yet from which deaf people had been excluded. Defining them as a minority underserved by essential health care services made minority-specific genetic counselling thus appear like a matter of equality and democracy.

Both developments – the refashioning of genetic counselling towards middle-class sensitivities and psychosocial research into disability – fostered new forms of cooperation between professionals, patients, and their families. In the spirit of community psychiatry, the NYSPI project, for example, promoted collaboration with the New York State deaf community – an exchange that changed professional perceptions of deafness and deaf people. Working with well-organized New York State deaf organizations and their self-confident leaders, the NYSPI developed a definition of deafness as a potentially stress-inducing condition, and the deaf as an overall well-adjusted social minority. For deaf community leaders – who had initiated the project in first place – working with the NYSPI was an opportunity to improve health care and rehabilitation services. Incorporating a growing number of young deaf professionals, the project blurred the line the line between hearing professionals and deaf service recipients or objects of research.

In various combinations, these trends – a more psychosocial approach to disability and difference, non-directive genetic counselling, a growing interest in deaf culture and sign language, and an ever more refined, yet far from complete understanding of genetic mechanisms – determined genetic deafness research in the 1970s and 1980s, although in a more explicitly political form. Increasingly, hearing professionals acted as intermediaries between the hearing and deaf worlds, popularizing ASL, Deaf culture, and community. This, in itself, was a remarkable development, given the strict dividing line hearing professionals long maintained towards deaf people. It is telling for the attraction of psychosocial models of difference, of ideals of justice and equality in engaging with minorities. To be sure, these engagements between predominantly middle-class professionals and predominantly middle-class community leaders produced often very static definitions of minority that could reinforce bias and preconceptions as much as erode them.

The 1970s campaign to eradicate Usher syndrome serves as a reminder that advocacy for one group can go hand in hand with ableist assumptions about another. McCay Vernon simultaneously defined deaf people as one of America's oppressed minorities and described deaf-blindness as a fate of suffering and deprivation. Here, promoting de-individualized eugenic measures could coexist with advocacy for Deaf culture, identity, and sign language – at least until deaf-blind individuals questioned narrow hearing-sighted perspectives. Emphasizing ability and autonomy, they challenged established narratives of suffering and defect. Professionals and deaf-blind people found a common denominator in shifting the debate from the genetic to the socioemotional risks associated with Usher syndrome. The motives of exclusion and endangered selfhood dominated 1980s discourse of Usher syndrome, although it could be cast as a clinical description of loss, or as a universal human search for belonging and fulfilment. The story of people with Usher syndrome also reminds us that genetic deafness is not one single condition, but encompasses a wide variety of identities and physical-sensory constellations. In future research, this variety and its overlap with race, gender, and different forms of disability deserves more attention.

Looking at the growing attractiveness of sign language and Deaf culture on the one hand, and debates over non-directive counselling on the other, it is not so surprising that geneticists such as Nance, Boughman, and Arnos began to seriously engage with deaf people's perspectives, values, and linguistic preferences. Their working towards ASL-based, culturally sensitive genetic counselling culminated with the establishment of the Gallaudet Genetic Services Center in 1984. In turn, Gallaudet and the Medical College of Virginia (MCV) genetics department – headed by Nance until 2002 – became centres of transmission, where scientists learned about Deaf culture and culturally sensitive genetic counselling. Arti Pandya, for example, professor of genetics and metabolism at the University of Chapel Hill, originally 'viewed hearing loss with a medical lens, considering it a disorder'. Yet as she joined Nance's department at MCV, and began working with Arnos at Gallaudet, she 'realized that ours was an extremely narrow view'. This discovery motivated her to 'delve deeper to understand their attitudes and the impact that discoveries in the genetics of hearing loss has on the Deaf community at large'. Pandya has since worked with Arnos on studies that explore the attitudes of d/Deaf people towards genetic counselling.[4]

For others, the influence of the Gallaudet/MCV group was more indirect. When University of California, Los Angeles (UCLA) genetic counsellor Christina Palmer began providing genetic testing and counselling for deafness in the early 2000s, she came into contact with California Deaf communities. Wanting to learn more about her clients, she contacted the Deaf studies department at California State University, Northridge and was referred to ASL scholar Patrick Boudreault. They decided to collaborate to provide culturally sensitive counselling for deaf people at UCLA, and to explore the attitudes of deaf people towards genetic testing. Boudreault's insight and insider knowledge, Palmer commented, was invaluable for her as a hearing person, the 'reason, really, why we were so successful with that project'.[5] When they began their work, they contacted Arnos for advice and training and profited from the Genetic Services Center's experience. In another project, Palmer and Boudreault collaborated to provide bilingual cancer genetics education in ASL and English to the Deaf community. Here, again, it was no longer deafness per se that was targeted; it was merely the uniting characteristic of a population at risk of other conditions – cancer here or mental illness at the NYSPI – that affect deaf or hearing people alike.[6]

More generally, within the relatively small field of genetic deafness research, the model of culturally sensitive counselling has been influential. Most American literature today at least acknowledges the existence of Deaf identities. The 2014 National Center of Biotechnology Information (NCBI) *Gene Review on Deafness and Hereditary Hearing Loss*, for example, gives an overview of several hundred forms of genetic deafness, alongside a discussion of diagnosis, treatment, and management. It also points to the existence of the American Deaf community with their 'unique social and societal attributes'. Deaf people, the authors explain, 'may view deafness as a distinguishing characteristic and not as a handicap, impairment, or medical condition requiring a "treatment" or "cure," or as something to be "prevented"'. They note that efficient communication requires a skilled interpreter, and that the 'use of certain terms is preferred', e.g. 'probability or chance versus risk' and that terms 'such as "affected," "abnormal," and "disease-causing" should be avoided'. Echoing Arnos, they caution that deaf people often look for genetic information for reasons other than 'prevention, reproduction, and family planning', and that it is thus important for the counsellor to inquire about individual concerns.[7]

Without a question, the projects described here have equalized and expanded deaf people's access to health care services and information. They are driven by a genuine belief in the need for exchange between client and professional, and in the right of minorities to their own culture and identity. At the same time, questions of race, class, and disability have been mostly absent from discussions about genetic services for deaf people. Like in other fields of science and medicine, genetics professionals tended to interact and identify mainly with those community members who share their own, usually white, middle-class values and background. Vice versa, deaf community leaders have long been white, male, and able-bodied. The very attempt, then, to diversify genetics by adopting the values of a minority community can also perpetuate patterns of bias and exclusion within this minority. As the study of intersectional identities is growing in Deaf and disability studies, these dimensions need to be incorporated more closely by medical service providers.

The politics and goals of genetics remain a much-discussed topic. Non-directive genetic counselling has often been cast as neutral and apolitical, and thus as safely removed from eugenic abuses. Yet the very attempt to distance oneself from political abuse has always been deeply political, too. The eugenicists of the first part of the century legitimized their work with the goal of improving race and humankind. By the end of the twentieth century, geneticists found justification in a different political ideology. Aligning themselves with deaf people's struggle for equality and diversity (usually white middle-class) geneticists portrayed themselves as advocates for a more just health care system accessible to neglected, underserved populations. This narrative turned geneticists into the vanguard of social progress, ahead of other professionals who were still tangled in bias and discrimination. Thus, if a deaf client expressed a wish for a deaf child, this was no longer to be seen as deviant and pathological. Rather, it had become a testing case for the much-discussed dogma of genetic counselling: non-directiveness. This move, however, may turn non-directiveness into an absolute value that cannot not be criticized without, simultaneously, criticizing the ideal of a diverse and tolerant society.

When, in the 1980s and 1990s, the Gallaudet Genetic Services Center claimed genetic knowledge to be empowering, this read very differently from early twentieth-century dreams of eugenic prevention. Yet there are important continuities in these changes. Various forms of genetic essentialism are one such continuity. Debates over the meaning of genetics are often reduced to questions of nature or nurture, that is, of genetic determinism versus sociocultural influences. It is a striking feature of genetic deafness research that for most of the actors in this book this was not true or relevant. For most professionals, genetics was just one element in a larger project of managing deafness. It was essential for navigating life, yet not necessarily a deterministic factor. This belief in the essentiality of genetic knowledge was something that hearing professionals – educators, eugenicists and geneticists, psychologists or psychiatrists – and, indeed, some d/Deaf or deaf-blind people shared. What, exactly, genetic awareness meant, however, could differ significantly, ranging from an instrument for achieving normalcy to a symbol of Deaf difference.

Such genetic essentialism rests on a compelling narrative, in which geneticists are the arbiters of an apparently natural progression from ignorance to enlightenment. Knowledge, here, always trumps ignorance. Yet this is not always the case, as has become apparent in debates over genetic testing for Chorea Huntington's disease or breast cancer. Some people with parents affected by Chorea Huntington's decide to forego genetic testing, even though they have a 50 per cent chance of having the disease themselves. A test would provide certain knowledge, yet some believe that it is less emotionally damaging not to know than to be certain to develop a debilitating and eventually fatal condition. With genetic testing for breast cancer, risk, certainty, and insecurity are distributed differently. A positive test for a BRCA 1 or 2 mutation means a high chance, yet no certainty, of developing breast cancer.[8] Despite such weighing of pros and cons, however, the right not to know is usually in the defensive. In an age of information technology and supposed self-determination, not knowing is considered quaint at best, if not a sign of unenlightened backwardness, endangering oneself and one's descendants.

The need to pursue genetic awareness might seem self-evident to us now, steeped as we are in the omnipresent rhetoric of genetic identity. Yet we should not take it as a given. The idea that genetics is part of our selfhood is a recent construction, tied to modern and postmodern ideas about identity and society. Capitalist consumerism and the ideals of liberal citizenship, historians have pointed out, created an identity culture in which self-achievement and self-improvement are desired life goals. And the psycho-sciences, Nicolas Rose has further argued, have promoted the notion of a hidden, true self that requires constant management under professional surveillance. This larger social trend for self-awareness, self-realization, and self-improvement has been central in creating the appeal of late twentieth-century individualized genetics, with its promise of improvement and of learning about our true selves.[9]

If we look back at perceptions of (genetic) deafness throughout the twentieth-century, there is a progression from understanding it as an innate disability to be overcome to something that is negotiated between individual and society, and thus culturally and socially constructed. By the early 2000s, however, this sociocultural framework no longer seems to be enough. There is an apparent need to fortify identity, ethnicity, and belonging with more biologistic-essentialist claims. In Deaf studies and history, too, claims about Deaf people's minority status – indeed, their ethnicity – have come to be supported by explicitly genetic claims. In 2000, for example, hearing psychologist Harlan Lane, and hearing psychiatrist Richard Pillard (both long-time advocates for Deaf culture) traced the genealogies of several multiple-generation deaf families back to the eighteenth and nineteenth centuries. They argue that 'a difference in the genetic basis' has influenced the development of Deaf identities and communities. Thus, a dominant pattern of inheritance produces families with deaf members in each generation who pass on their language and values. With recessive pattern, on the other hand, deafness is rarer and might skip a generation. Producing only isolated deaf individuals, recessive inheritance supported assimilation to hearing society and hindered the creation of a Deaf 'class consciousness'.[10] Lane and Pillard's 2011 *The People of the Eye: Deaf Ethnicity and Ancestry*, written together with Gallaudet archivist Ulf Hedberg, rehearses these theories within a more explicitly ethnographic framework.[11]

Grounding culture in biology, others have evoked biocultural diversity; a term that is as vaguely defined as politically attractive. In the introduction to the 2014 essay collection *Deaf Gain: Raising the Stakes for Human Diversity*, Gallaudet Deaf studies scholars Joseph Murray and H.-Dirksen Bauman write that 'the gene [sic] for deafness has stubbornly persisted over thousands of generations'; proof that 'deafness is not an evolutionary error but a natural human variation that continues to thrive'.[12] In the same volume, historian David Armstrong point to the specific evolutionary value of sign languages to support the notion of Deaf gain, the idea that Deafness and Deaf people contribute positively to the variety of human experience.[13] Certainly, this turn towards biological essentialism is not limited to the Deaf community. The rapidly rising popularity of neurodiversity provides another influential example. Initially advocated as a more positive, enabling definition of autism, neurodiversity now has reached a much wider popular and scientific valence. Advocates, but also scientists, have used neurodiversity for explaining differences in behaviour or personality not as social deviance, but as immutable – and valuable – neurological differences, expressions of human diversity.[14] There lurks, then, underneath these important celebrations of human difference, the old pressure to prove one's value to society, whether it is in terms of contributing to the human gene pool or economic productivity.

There are two ways of understanding this tendency to locate identity, belonging, and, once more, social value in supposedly innate, embodied, and unchangeable dimensions – be it brain or genes. One is more critical, the other more affirmative or celebratory. Disability and Deaf scholars and activists tend towards the affirmative. They celebrate (their own) genetic or neurological selfhood as a successful assertion of autonomy and agency; as a re-appropriation of knowledge from the scientific regime of normalcy; and as a celebration of human (bio)diversity. Historians and sociologists of science and medicine, on the other hand, have pointed to the close ties between notions of biodiverse selfhood and biomedical citizenship. They argue that by focusing more and more on disease prevention, modern biomedicine has turned us all into potential patients, more or less at risk of a wide range of conditions, from cancer to dementia. This constant at-risk status dissolves the old dichotomy of sick and healthy, and, to an extent, of normal and pathological. Instead, we are supposed to internalize a medicalized lifestyle that is supposed to keep these risks at bay. Genetic deafness research provides a good example for this development. Where once it was only the deaf individual who was considered at risk of passing on deafness, this risk expanded to hearing family members, too, and soon to the population at large, who all might carry genes for deafness. Likewise, where once a deaf person was only assessed for their risk of passing on hearing loss, now a genetic assessment encompasses a myriad of other, connected or unconnected conditions.[15]

In talking about genetic or neurological selfhood we have, then, one narrative that reaffirms the absolutizing power of science and medicine, and another that celebrates the re-appropriation of knowledge by individuals with disability/difference. Both interpretations, however, rest on the belief that these identities and ideologies are recent developments. They suggest a tripartite periodization: a medical-eugenic era with professionals dominating definitions of pathology and normalcy; a period of cultural relativism and social activism during the 1960s, 1970s and 1980s; and an era of actor-driven bio-identities and (bio)diversity, in which we live presently. This, I believe, obscures important continuities that become apparent when we move away from a strict separation of science and social activism. Scientists and physicians, of course, have always been involved in politics and social movements. Eugenicists often were zealous social reformers, engaged in a variety of agendas from all over the political spectrum. Yet from mid-century on, I have traced a different form of social advocacy that rested on a merger of biological essentialism and cultural relativism. NYSPI scientists in the 1950s and 1960s, McCay Vernon in the 1970s and 1980, and, later, Nance, Boughman, and Arnos aligned with adult communities that asserted their sociocultural difference with growing confidence and success. In a period, in which the authority of science and medicine became increasingly challenged, these collaborations provided new professional roles. Here, the scientific experts saw themselves as an ally to minorities in their struggles for equality and acceptance.

Throughout the twentieth century and into the twenty-first, genetic counselling has been an enterprise of education and persuasion, of convincing deaf people that knowing one's genetic make-up is essential for navigating life. At least since the 1960s, this was no longer simply a process in which hearing scientists imposed their values and norms on deaf objects, but an exchange in which deaf or deaf-blind people – clients, lay people, or professionals themselves – inserted their own ideas about the meaning of genes and heredity. Sometimes, they rejected genetic knowledge and awareness as irrelevant or restricting. At other times, they accepted or embraced genetics as an important part of their identity, or as a useful rhetorical tool. Certainly, when some Deaf activists now claim Deaf (deaf?) people to be an ethnogenetic group of shared ancestry, this is an act of re-appropriating genetic knowledge in a society that still, predominantly, sees such genes as a defect. Yet the roots for this ethnobiological identity politics also share a longer history of geneticists propagating genetic knowledge as essential self-knowledge, and encouraging genetic awareness as a form of political empowerment.

Notes

1 Nance, 'The genetics of deafness', 109, 118. Gallaudet philosopher Theresa Blankmeyer-Burke believes, on the contrary, that the 'ethical issues of cochlear implant surgery seem almost quaint and outmoded' compared to genetic technology, which she sees as the 'newest potential threat to the continued existence of the Deaf community'. See T. Blankmeyer-Burke, 'Quest for a deaf child: ethics and genetics' (PhD dissertation, University of New Mexico, 2011), p. 8. Also see J. Murray, 'Genetics: a future peril facing the global deaf community', in H. Goodstein, *The Deaf Way II Reader: Perspectives from the Second International Conference on Deaf Culture* (Washington, DC: Gallaudet University Press, 2006), pp. 351–6.

2 For the history of and controversies around CIs see S. S. Blume, *The Artificial Ear: Cochlear Implants and the Culture of Deafness* (New Brunswick, NJ: Rutgers University Press, 2010); L. Mauldin, *Made to Hear: Cochlear Implants and Raising Deaf Children* (London: University of Minnesota Press, 2016).

3 Blankmeyer-Burke has covered this case most extensively, and provides a detailed analysis of the bioethical issues at stake in the use of genetic technology. See Blankmeyer-Burke, 'Quest for a deaf child'.

4 See Anon., 'Meet Dr. Arti Pandya, UNC Children's chief of genetics and metabolism', *UNC's Children News, Care* 2 (2015), http://news.unchealthcare.org/unc-childrens/news/care-2015/issue-2/genetics [accessed 20 September 2018]. For her work with Arnos see e.g. P. R. Taneja, A. Pandya, D. L. Foley, L. V. Niceley, and K. S. Arnos, 'Attitudes of deaf individuals towards genetic testing', *American Journal of Medical Genetics Part A*, 130A:1 (2004), 17–21.

5 'Oral history interview with Christina Palmer', Los Angeles, CA, 13 August 2013. Interviewer: Marion Schmidt.

6 Ibid., 9–10, 19–20. For research on attitudes towards genetic testing see e.g. P. Boudreault, C. Palmer, et al., 'Deaf adults' reasons for genetic testing depend on cultural affiliation: results from a prospective, longitudinal genetic counseling and testing study', *Journal of Deaf Studies and Deaf Education*, 15:3 (2010), 209–27.

7 Shearer et al., 'Deafness and hereditary hearing loss overview'.

8 For Chorea Huntington see Wexler, *Mapping Fate*; K. A. Quaid, 'A few words from a 'wise' woman', in R. F. Weir, S. C. Lawrence, and E. Fales (eds), *Genes and Human Self-knowledge: Historical and Philosophical Reflections on Modern Genetics* (Iowa City: University of Iowa Press, 1994), pp. 2–17. For a discussion of risk and breast cancer see Klawiter, *Biopolitics of Breast Cancer*.

9 See e.g. Rose, *Governing the Soul*. For genetics in particular see e.g. Weir, Lawrence, and Fales (eds), *Genes and Human Self-Knowledge*.

10 H. L. Lane, R. Pillard, and M. French, 'Origins of the American Deaf-world: assimilating and differentiating societies and their relation to genetic patterning', *Sign Language Studies*, 1:1 (2000), 17–44, here 37.

11 H. L. Lane, R. Pillard, and U. Hedberg, *The People of the Eye: Deaf Ethnicity and*

Ancestry (New York: Oxford University Press, 2011). For other reflections on deaf ethnicity see e.g. R. C. Eckert, 'Deafnicity: a study of strategic and adaptive responses to audism by members of the deaf American community of Culture' (PhD dissertation, University of Michigan, 2005).

12 H.-D. Bauman and J. J. Murray, 'Deaf gain: an introduction', in H.-D. Bauman and J. J. Murray (eds), *Deaf Gain: Raising the Stakes for Human Diversity* (Minneapolis, MN: University of Minnesota Press, 2014), pp. xv–xiii, here pp. xix–xx.

13 D. Armstrong, 'Deaf gain in evolutionary perspective', in Bauman and Murray (eds), *Deaf Gain*, pp. 77–94.

14 See e.g. N. Bagatell, 'From cure to community: transforming notions of autism', *Ethos*, 38:1 (2010), 33–55; S. Silberman, *NeuroTribes: The Legacy of Autism and the Future of Neurodiversity* (New York: Avery, 2016); J. Singer, *Neurodiversity: The Birth of an Idea* (Lexington, KY, 2017); J. den Houting, 'Neurodiversity: an insider's perspective', *Autism*, 23:2 (2019), 271–3. For a more general analysis of recent neuro-scientific discourse see e.g. S. Maasen and B. Sutter (eds), *On Willing Selves: Neoliberal Politics Vis-à-Vis the Neuroscientific Challenge* (Basingstoke: Palgrave Macmillan, 2007); F. Vidal and F. Ortega, *Being Brains: Making the Cerebral Subject* (New York: Fordham University Press, 2017).

15 For theories of biomedicine and biomedical citizenship see Lock and Nguyen, *An Anthropology of Biomedicine*; for identity politics and genetics e.g. K. Schramm, D. Skinner, and R. Rottenburg (eds), *Identity Politics and the New Genetics: Re/creating Categories of Difference and Belonging* (New York: Berghahn Books, 2012). For a more general take on disability and biocultural diversity see e.g. L. J. Davis, *The End of Normal: Identity in a Biocultural Era* (Ann Arbor, MI: University of Michigan Press, 2013).

Bibliography

Interviews

'Oral history interview with Walter Nance', Sewanee, TN, 11 September 2006. Interviewer: Nathaniel Comfort. UCLA-Johns Hopkins Oral History of Human Genetics Project.

'Oral history interview with Kathleen Shaver Arnos', Washington, DC, 9 October 2012. Interviewer: Marion Schmidt.

'Oral history interview with Christina Palmer', Los Angeles, CA, 13 August 2013. Interviewer: Marion Schmidt.

'Oral history interview with Joann Boughman', Adelphi, MD, 27 August 2013. Interviewer: Marion Schmidt.

'Oral history interview with Kenneth Z. Altshuler', Dallas/Baltimore, 6 February 2014. Interviewer: Marion Schmidt.

Archival material

Eskind Biomedical Library Special Collections, Vanderbilt University Medical Center, Nashville, TN, Anne J. Sweeney Papers.

Gallaudet University Archives, Departmental Files, Box 28, Folder 99.1, 'Genetic Services Center, Brochures', n.d.

Gallaudet University Archives, Departmental Files, Folder 35, File 72.1, 'Office of Demographic Studies Reports', 1977 (No. 1).

Gallaudet University Archives, Manuscript Collection, MSS 166, Levine, Edna Simon, 'Biographical Sketch, Edna Simon Levine'.

Gallaudet University Archives, Manuscript Collection, MSS 166, Levine, Edna Simon, Box 15, Folder 22, draft proposal, undated [c. 1953] 'Mental Health project for the deaf, objectives and progress reports'.

Gallaudet University Archives, Manuscript Collection, MSS 166, Levine, Edna Simon, Box 4, Folder 14, Correspondence Department of Health, Education and Welfare, 'OVR Press release', 25 March 1955, p. 1.

Gallaudet University Archives, Manuscript Collection, MSS 166, Levine, Edna Simon, Box 21, Folder 31, 'Speeches, Mental Health Center for the Deaf', April 1958.

Gallaudet University Archives, Manuscript Collection, MSS 166, Levine, Edna Simon Box 5, Folder 49, correspondence Kallmann Franz J., 'Levine to Kallmann', 17 December 1962.

Gallaudet University Archives, MSS 048, Vernon, McCay, Box 5, Folders 22 and 23, McCay Vernon, correspondence 'Usher syndrome' (1966–1974).

Special Collections and University Archives, UMass Amherst Libraries, Clarke School for the Deaf (MS 742), 'Biographical file, Hopkins, Louise Alice'.

Special Collections and University Archives, UMass Amherst Libraries, Clarke School for the Deaf (MS 742), 'Biographical file Ruth Guilder'.

University Archives, Kenneth Spencer Research Library, University of Kansas, Personal papers of Fritz Heider, 'First impressions of Clarke School', Fritz Heider collection, PP. 343, Box 26, Folder 25.

Published sources

Adorno, T. W., E. Frenkel-Brunswik, D. J. Levinson, and N. Sanford, *The Authoritarian Personality* (New York: Harper, 1950).

Allen, G. E., 'The Eugenics Record Office at Cold Spring Harbor, 1910–1940: an essay in institutional history', *Osiris 2nd series*, 2 (1986), 225–64.

Altshuler, K. Z., 'Sexual patterns and relationships', in J. D. Rainer, K. Z. Altshuler, and F. J. Kallmann (eds), *Family and Mental Health Problems in a Deaf Population* (New York: New York State Psychiatric Unit, 1963), pp. 92–112.

Altshuler, K. Z., 'The psychiatric preventive programs in a school for the deaf', in Rainer and Altshuler (eds), *Psychiatry and the Deaf* (1968), pp. 11–23.

Altshuler, K. Z. and G. S. Baroff, 'Educational background and vocational adjustment', in Rainer, Altshuler, and Kallmann (eds), *Family and Mental Health* (1963), pp. 116–30.

Altshuler, K. Z., G. S. Baroff, and J. D. Rainer, 'Operational description of pilot clinic', in Rainer, Altshuler, and Kallmann (eds), *Family and Mental Health* (1963), pp. 155–66.

Anderson, R. J., C. E. Keller, and J. M. Karp, *Enhancing Diversity: Educators With Disabilities* (Washington, DC: Gallaudet University Press, 1998).

Annala, L., 'Facing the future with Usher Syndrome', in N. L. Tully (ed.), *Papers presented at Workshop on Usher's Syndrome, December 2–3, 1976. Conducted by Helen Keller National Center for Deaf-Blind Youths and Adults* (Sands Point, NY: Helen Keller National Center, 1977), pp. 19–22.

Anon., 'Chin Sik Chung', *American Men & Women of Science: A Biographical Directory of Today's Leaders in Physical, Biological, and Related Sciences.* (Detroit, MI: Gale, 2008), www.gale.com/uk/c/biography-in-context [accessed 4 July 2015].

Anon., 'Edna Simon Levine', *Contemporary Authors Online* (Detroit, MI: Gale, 2008), www.gale.com/uk/c/biography-in-context [accessed 4 July 2015].

Anon., 'Kenneth Stephen Brown', *American Men & Women of Science: A Biographical Directory of Today's Leaders in Physical, Biological, and Related Sciences* (Detroit: Gale, 2008), www.gale.com/uk/c/biography-in-context [accessed 4 July 2015].

Anon., 'Meet Dr. Arti Pandya, UNC Children's chief of genetics and metabolism', *UNC's Children News, Care* 2 (2015), http://news.unchealthcare.org/uncchildrens/news/care-2015/issue-2/genetics [accessed 20 September 2018].

Anon., 'Obituaries. Jerome D. Schein', *The Hearing Journal*, 63:6 (June 2010), 56.

Anon., 'Ruth Hudgins, 101, teacher, music lover', *Daily Hampshire Gazette* (April 29 2009).

Armstrong, D., 'Deaf gain in evolutionary perspective', in H.-D. Bauman and J. J. Murray (eds), *Deaf Gain: Raising the Stakes for Human Diversity* (Minneapolis, MN: University of Minnesota Press, 2014), pp. 77–94.

Armstrong, D. F., *The History of Gallaudet University: 150 years of a Deaf American Institution* (Washington DC: Gallaudet University Press, 2014).

Arnos, K. S., 'The implications of genetic testing for deafness', *Ear and Hearing*, 24:4 (2003), 324–31.

Arnos, K. S., 'Attitudes of deaf individuals towards genetic testing', *American Journal of Medical Genetics*, 130:17 (2004), 17–21.

Arnos, K. S., J. Israel, and M. Cunningham, 'Genetic counselling of the deaf', *Annals of the New York Academy of Sciences*, 630 (1991), 212–22.

Arnos, K. S., M. Cunningham, J. Israel, and M. L. Marazita, 'Innovative approach to genetic counseling services for the deaf population', *American Journal of Medical Genetics*, 44 (1992), 345–51.

Arthur, L. J., 'Some hereditary syndromes that include deafness', *Developmental Medicine and Child Neurology*, 7:4 (1966), 395–409.

Bagatell, N., 'From cure to community: transforming notions of autism', *Ethos*, 38:1 (2010), 33–55.

Baldwin, S. C., *Pictures in the Air: The Story of the National Theatre of the Deaf* (Washington, DC: Galludet University Press, 1998).

Barnartt, S. N. and R. K. Scotch, *Disability Protests: Contentious Politics 1970–1999* (Washington, DC: Gallaudet University Press, 2001).

Barnes, C. and G. Mercer, *Independent Futures: Creating User-Led Disability Services in a Disabling Society* (Bristol: Policy Press, 2006).

Baroff, G. S., 'Patterns of socialization and community integration', in Rainer, Altshuler, and Kallmann (eds), *Family and Mental Health* (1963), pp. 113–15.

Bauman, H.-D. and J. J. Murray, 'Deaf gain: an introduction', in Bauman and Murray (eds), *Deaf Gain* (2014), pp. xv–xiii.

Baynton, D. C., '"A silent exile on this earth": the metaphorical construction of deafness in the 19th century', *American Quarterly*, 44 (1992), 216–43.

Baynton, D. C., *Forbidden Signs: American Culture and the Campaign against Sign Language* (Chicago, IL: University of Chicago Press, 1998).

Baynton, D. C., '"These pushful days": time and disability in the age of eugenics', *Health and History*, 13:2 (2011), 43–64.

Bell, A. G., *Memoir Upon the Formation of a Deaf Variety of the Human Race* (Washington, DC: U.S. Government Printing Office, 1884), http://catalog.hathitrust.org/api/volumes/oclc/2141276.html [accessed 16 October 2019].

Bell, A. G., *A Few Thoughts Concerning Eugenics* (Washington, DC: Judd & Detweiler, 1908).

Bess, F. H. (ed.), *Childhood Deafness: Causation, Assessment, and Management* (New York: Grune & Stratton, 1977).

Best, H., *The Deaf: Their Position in Society and the Provision for their Education in the United States* (New York: T. Y. Crowell Co., 1914).

Best, H., *The Deaf-Mute Population of the United States, 1920: A Statistical Analysis of the Data Obtained at the Fourteenth Decentennial Census* (Washington, DC: U.S. Government Printing Office, 1928).

Bieber, F. R., 'Genetic studies of questionnaire data from a residential school for the deaf' (PhD dissertation, Virginia Commonwealth University, 1981).

Bieber, F. R. and W. E. Nance, 'Hereditary hearing loss', in L. G. Jackson and R. N. Schimke (eds), *Clinical Genetics: A Source Book for Physicians* (New York: Wiley, 1979), pp. 443–61.

Bix, A. S., 'Experiences and voices of eugenics field-workers: "women's work" in biology', *Social Studies of Science*, 27:4 (1997), 625–68.

Blankmeyer-Burke, T., 'Quest for a deaf child: ethics and genetics' (PhD dissertation, University of New Mexico, 2011).

Blume, S. S., *The Artificial Ear: Cochlear Implants and the Culture of Deafness* (New Brunswick, NJ: Rutgers University Press, 2010).

Boltseridge, N. H., 'Identical confusion: the history of twin studies on sexual orientation 1952–1973' (MA thesis, Oregon State University, 2004).

Boudreault, P., C. Palmer, et al., 'Deaf adults' reasons for genetic testing depend on cultural affiliation: results from a prospective, longitudinal genetic counseling and testing study', *Journal of Deaf Studies and Deaf Education*, 15:3 (2010), 209–27.

Boughman, J. A., 'Population genetic studies of retinitis pigmentosa' (PhD dissertation, Indiana University, 1978).

Boughman, J. A. and K. A. Shaver, 'Responsibilities in genetic counseling for the deaf', *American Journal of Human Genetics*, 35:6 (1983), 1317–19.

Branson, J. and D. Miller, *Damned for Their Difference: The Cultural Construction of Deaf People as Disabled: A Sociological History* (Washington, DC: Gallaudet University Press, 2002).

Brewer, G. D. and J. S. Kakalis, *Serving the Deaf-Blind Population: Planning for 1980* (Santa Monica, CA: Rand Corp, 1974).

Brown, T. M., '"Stress" in US wartime psychiatry: World War II and the immediate aftermath', in D. Cantor (ed.), *Stress, Shock, and Adaptation in the Twentieth Century* (Rochester, NY: University of Rochester Press, 2014), pp. 121–41.

Burch, S., *Signs of Resistance: American Deaf Cultural History, 1900 to World War II* (New York: New York University Press, 2002).

Burch, S. and A. Kafer (eds), *Deaf and Disability Studies: Interdisciplinary Perspectives* (Washington, DC: Gallaudet University Press, 2010).

Callahan, R. E., *Education and the Cult of Efficiency: A Study of the Social forces that Have Shaped the Administration of the Public Schools* (Chicago, IL: University of Chicago Press, 1962).

Carey, A. C., *On the Margins of Citizenship: Intellectual Disability and Civil Rights in Twentieth-Century America* (Philadelphia, PA: Temple University Press, 2010).

Chadarevian, S. de, *Designs for Life: Molecular Biology after World War II* (Cambridge: Cambridge University Press, 2002).

Christensen, D., '"In a glass box": Clarke School for the Deaf alumni detail decades

of abuse', *Daily Hampshire Gazette*, 1 January 2019, www.gazettenet.com/Clarke-School-alumni-detail-abuse-they-suffered-19985099 [accessed 29 May 2019].
Chung, C. S. and K. S. Brown, 'Family studies of early childhood deafness ascertained through the Clarke School for the Deaf', *American Journal of Human Genetics*, 22:6 (1970), 630–44.
Chung, C. S., O. W. Robinson, and N. E. Morton, 'A note on deaf mutism', *Annals of Human Genetics*, 23 (1959), 357–66.
Clark, H. D., 'We are the same but different: navigating African American and deaf cultural identities' (PhD dissertation, University of Washington, 2010).
Clark, J. L., *Where I Stand: On the Signing Community and My Deafblind Experience* (Minneapolis, MN: Handtype Press, 2014).
Clarke School for the Deaf, *A Child at the Clarke School for the Deaf* (Northampton, MA: Clarke School for the Deaf, 1927).
Clarke School for the Deaf, *The Coolidge Fund for the Clarke School and the Deaf* (New York: Coolidge Fund, 1929).
Cohen, M. M., G. Cassady, and B. L. Hanna, 'A genetic study of hereditary renal dysfunction with associated nerve deafness', *American Journal of Human Genetics*, 13:4 (1961), 379–89.
Comfort, N. C., '"Polyhybrid heterogeneous bastards": promoting medical genetics in America in the 1930s and 1940s', *Journal of the History of Medicine and Allied Sciences*, 61 (2006), 415–55.
Comfort, N. C., *The Science of Human Perfection: How Genes Became the Heart of American Medicine* (New Haven, CT: Yale University Press, 2012).
Conrad, P., *The Medicalization of Society: On the Transformation of Human Conditions into Treatable Disorders* (Baltimore, MD: Johns Hopkins University Press, 2007).
Cottebrune, A., 'Franz Josef Kallmann (1897–1965) und der Transfer psychiatrisch-genetischer Wissenschaftskonzepte vom NS-Deutschland in die U.S.A', *Medizinhistorisches Journal*, 44:3–4 (2009), 296–324.
Cowan, R. S., *Heredity and Hope: The Case for Genetic Screening* (Cambridge, MA: Harvard University Press, 2008).
Crowe, S. J. and J. W. Baylor, 'The prevention of deafness', *Journal of the American Medical Association*, 112:7 (1939), 585–90.
Davenport, C. B. and M. Steggerda, *Race Crossing in Jamaica* (Washington, DC: Carnegie Institution of Washington, 1929).
Davis, K., *The Making of Our Bodies, Ourselves: How Feminism Travels Across Borders* (Durham, NC: Duke University Press, 2007).
Davis, L. J., *Enforcing Normalcy: Disability, Deafness, and the Body* (London: Verso, 1995).
Davis, L. J., 'Introduction: disability, normality, and power', in L. J. Davis (ed.), *The Disability Studies Reader* (London and New York: Routledge, 2012), pp. 1–17.
Davis, L. J., *The End of Normal: Identity in a Biocultural Era* (Ann Arbor, MI: University of Michigan Press, 2013).

Day, C. W., 'Current screening procedures for the Usher syndrome at residential schools for the deaf', *American Annals of the Deaf*, 127:1 (1982), 45–8.

Den Houting, J., 'Neurodiversity: an insider's perspective', *Autism*, 23:2 (2019), 271–3.

Division of Research, Gallaudet College, 'Proposal: Demonstration of an Innovative Approach to Genetic Counseling Services for the Deaf Population to Department of Health and Human Services Bureau of Health Care Delivery and Assistance Division of Maternal and Child Health 5600 Fishers Lange Rockville, Maryland 20857 by Division of Research, Gallaudet College' (Gallaudet College, Washington, DC: Division of Research, May 1 1984).

Dowbiggin, I. R., *The Sterilization Movement and Global Fertility in the Twentieth Century* (New York: Oxford University Press, 2008).

Driggs, F., 'The causes of deafness', *Volta Review*, 15 (1913), 330–4.

Eckert, R. C., 'Deafnicity: a study of strategic and adaptive responses to audism by members of the Deaf American community of culture' (PhD dissertation, University of Michigan, 2005).

Edwards, R. A. R., *Words Made Flesh: Nineteenth-Century Deaf Education and the Growth of Deaf Culture* (New York: New York University Press, 2014).

Edwards, T., 'Language emergence in the Seattle DeafBlind community' (PhD dissertation, University of California, 2014).

Eghigian, G., A. Killen, and C. Leuenberger (eds), *The Self as Project: Politics and the Human Sciences* (Chicago, IL: University of Chicago Press, 2007).

Ennis, W. T., 'Hereditarian ideas and eugenic ideals at the National Deaf-Mute College' (PhD dissertation, University of Iowa, 2015).

Erlenmeyer-Kimling, L., 'Medical genetics', in B. A. Fallon, J. M. Gorman, J. M. Oldham and H. Pardes (eds), *The New York State Psychiatric Institute: American Psychiatry at the Centennial 1896–1996* (New York: The New York State Psychiatric Institute, 1998), pp. 33–42.

Fay, E. A., *Marriages of the Deaf in America: An Inquiry Concerning the Results of Marriages of the Deaf in America* (Washington, DC: Gibson bros., printers and bookbinders, 1898).

Fisch, L., 'Syndromes and early detection of deafness', *Reports of the Proceedings of the International Congress of the Deaf and the Forty-First Meeting of the Convention of American Instructors of the Deaf, Gallaudet College, Washington D.C. June 22–28 1963* (Washington, DC: U.S. Government Printing Office, 1964), pp. 627–32.

Fleck, L., *Entstehung und Entwicklung einer Wissenschaftlichen Tatsache: Einführung in die Lehre vom Denkstil und Denkkollektiv* (Frankfurt am Main: Suhrkamp, 1980, first edition Basel: Benno Schwabe, 1935).

Fraser, G. R., *The Causes of Profound Deafness in Childhood: A Study of 3,535 Individuals with Severe Hearing Loss Present at Birth or of Childhood Onset* (Baltimore, MD: Johns Hopkins University Press, 1976).

Freeden, M., 'Eugenics and progressive thought: a study in ideological affinity', *Historical Journal*, 22 (1979), 645–71.

Friedman, F., N. Leeds, and A. Sussman, 'Adjustment problems of the Deaf: panel of deaf adults', in J. D. Rainer and K. Z. Altshuler (eds), *Psychiatry and the Deaf: Workshop for Psychiatrists on Extending Mental Health Services to the Deaf* (Washington, DC: U.S. Department of Health, Education, and Welfare, Social and Rehabilitation Service, 1968), pp. 25–36.

Gallaudet College, *Signs for Genetic Counseling: For Genetic Counselors, Clients, and Sign Language Interpreters* (Washington, DC: National Academy of Gallaudet College, 1983).

Gannon, J. R., J. Butler, and L.-J. Gilbert, *Deaf Heritage: A Narrative History of Deaf America* (Silver Spring, MD: National Association of the Deaf, 1981).

Gienow-McConnella, H., 'The story of Mr. and Mrs. Deaf: Deaf American historiography, past, present, and future', *Critical Disability Discourses/Discourse Critiques dans le Champ du Handicap*, 7 (2015), 109–44.

Gill, M. C., *Already Doing It: Intellectual Disability and Sexual Agency* (Minneapolis, MN: University of Minnesota Press, 2015).

Glass, B., 'In memoriam, Franz J. Kallmann', *Proceedings of the Annual Meeting of the American Psychopathological Association*, 55 (1967), 322–32.

Glover, J., *Choosing Children. Genes, Disability, and Design* (Oxford: Clarendon Press, 2006).

Goddard, H. H., *The Kallikak Family: A Study in the Heredity of Feeble-Mindedness* (New York: The Macmillan Company, 1912).

Goffman, E., *Stigma: Notes on the Management of Spoiled Identity* (Englewood Cliffs, NJ: Prentice-Hall, 1963).

Greenwald, B. H., 'Alexander Graham Bell through the lens of eugenics, 1883–1922' (doctoral dissertation, The George Washington University, 2002).

Grinker, R. R., 'Conference summary and comments', in Rainer and Altshuler (eds), *Psychiatry and the Deaf* (1968), pp. 147–53.

Grinker, R. R., *Psychiatric Diagnosis, Therapy, and Research on the Psychotic Deaf: Final Report, September 1, 1969* (Washington, DC: U.S. Department of Health, Education, and Welfare, Social Rehabilitation Service, Rehabilitation Services Administration, 1971).

Grob, G. N., *From Asylum to Community: Mental Health Policy in Modern America* (Princeton, NJ: Princeton University Press, 1992).

Grob, G. N., 'Creation of the National Institute of Mental Health'; *Public Health Reports*, 111:4 (1996), 378–81.

Groce, N. E., *Everyone Here Spoke Sign Language: Hereditary Deafness on Martha's Vineyard* (Cambridge, MA: Harvard University Press, 1987).

Hallgren, B., 'Retinitis pigmentosa in combination with congenital deafness and vestibulocerebellar ataxia; with psychiatric abnormality in some cases; a clinical and genetic study', *Acta Genetica et Statistica Medica*, 8:2 (1958), 97–104.

Halliwell, M., *Therapeutic Revolutions: Medicine, Psychiatry, and American culture, 1945–1970* (New Brunswick, NJ: Rutgers University Press, 2014).

Hammer, E., 'Needs of adolescents who have Usher's syndrome', *American Annals of the Deaf*, 123:3 (1978), 389–94.

Hannaway, C. and V. A. Harden, *Biomedicine in the Twentieth Century: Practices, Policies, and Politics* (Amsterdam: IOS Press, 2008).

Harmon, K. C., 'Growing up to become hearing: dreams of passing in oral deaf education', in J. A. Brune and D. J. Wilson (eds), *Disability and Passing: Blurring the Lines of Identity* (Philadelphia, PA: Temple University Press, 2013), pp. 167–98.

Harris, R. R., *Dental Science in a New Age: A History of the National Institute of Dental Research* (Rockville, MD: Montrose Press, 1989).

Harrod, M. J. E., 'Genetic counseling for Usher's syndrome patients and their families', in Tully (ed.), *Workshop on Usher's Syndrome* (1977), pp. 376–80.

Heider, F., *The Life of a Psychologist: An Autobiography* (Lawrence, KS: University Press of Kansas).

Heider, F. and G. M. Heider, *Studies in the Psychology of the Deaf, No. 2* (Evanston, IL: American Psychological Association, 1941).

Hodgson, K. W., *The Deaf and Their Problems: A Study in Special Education* (New York: Philosophical Library, 1954).

Hoffman, B. R., *Health Care for Some: Rights and Rationing in the United States since 1930* (Chicago, IL: University of Chicago Press, 2013).

Hopkins, L. A., 'The influence of the type of audiogram upon the child's ability to interpret speech sounds' (MS thesis, Massachusetts State College Amherst, 1939).

Hopkins, L. A., 'Studies on the inheritance of deafness in the pupils of the Clarke School for the Deaf: the collection of family histories, pedigrees and audiometer readings', *The Laryngoscope*, 56:10 (1946), 570–82.

Hopkins, L. A., 'Heredity and deafness', *Eugenics Quarterly*, 1:3 (1954), 193–9.

Hopkins, L. A. and R. P. Guilder, *Clarke School Studies Concerning the Heredity of Deafness: Pedigree Data 1930–1940* (Northampton, MA: Clarke School for the Deaf, 1949).

Hopkins, L. A. and L. G. Kinzer, 'Comparison of a group of rubella-deafened children with a group of hereditarily deaf children and their sibs', *American Journal of Diseases of Children*, 78:2 (1949), 182–200.

Hopkins, L. A. and R. Post, 'Deafmutism in two pairs of identical twins', *Journal of Heredity*, 47:2 (1956), 88–90.

Jankowski, K., *Deaf Empowerment: Emergence, Struggle, and Rhetoric* (Washington, DC: Gallaudet University Press, 2013).

Johnson, R. O., *Standardization, Efficiency, Heredity: Schools for the Deaf* (Indianapolis, IN: Burford, 1920).

Kallmann, F. J., 'Die Fruchtbarkeit der Schizophrenen', in H. Harmsen (ed.), *Bevölkerungsfragen: Bericht d. Internat. Kongresses f. Bevölkerungswissenschaft, Berlin, 26. Aug.–1. Sept. 1935* (Munich: J. F. Lehmanns Verlag, 1936), pp. 725–9.

Kallmann, F. J., *Heredity in Health and Mental Disorder: Principles of Psychiatric Genetics in the Light of Comparative Twin Studies* (New York: Norton, 1953).

Kallmann, F. J., 'Twin and sibship study of overt male homosexuality', *American Journal of Human Genetics*, 4:2 (1953), 136–46.

Kallmann, F. J., 'Genetic research and counseling in the mental health field, present and future', in F. J. Kallmann, L. Erlenmeyer-Kimling, E. V. Glanville, and J. D. Rainer (eds), *Expanding Goals of Genetics in Psychiatry: Anniversary Symposium of the Department of Medical Genetics, New York State Psychiatric Institute, October 27–28, 1961* (New York: Grune & Stratton, 1962), pp. 250–5.

Kallmann, F. J., 'Some genetic aspects of deafness and their implications for family counseling', in *Reports of the Proceedings of the International Congress of the Deaf and the Forty-First Meeting of the Convention of American Instructors of the Deaf, Gallaudet College, Washington D.C. June 22–28 1963* (Washington, DC: U.S. Government Printing Office, 1964), pp. 639–62.

Kelly, J. G., 'The National Institute of Mental Health and the founding of the field of community psychology', in W. E. Pickren and S. F. Schneider (eds), *Psychology and the National Institute of Mental Health: A Historical Analysis of Science, Practice, and Policy* (Washington, DC: American Psychological Association, 2005), pp. 233–60.

Kevles, D. J., *In the Name of Eugenics: Genetics and the Uses of Human Heredity: With a New Preface by the Author* (Cambridge, MA: Harvard University Press, 1997).

Kimmelman, B. A., 'The American Breeders' Association: genetics and eugenics in an agricultural context, 1903–13', *Social Studies of Science*, 13:2 (1983), 163–204.

Kinloch, G. C., *The Sociology of Minority Group Relations* (Englewood Cliffs, NJ: Prentice-Hall, 1979).

Klaber, M. and A. Falek, 'Delinquency and crime', in Rainer, Altshuler, and Kallmann (eds), *Family and Mental Health* (1963), pp. 141–51.

Klawiter, M., *The Biopolitics of Breast Cancer: Changing Cultures of Disease and Activism* (Minneapolis, MN: University of Minnesota Press, 2008).

Kline, W., *Building a Better Race: Gender, Sexuality, and Eugenics from the Turn of the Century to the Baby Boom* (Berkeley, CA: University of California Press, 2005).

Kloepfer, H. W., J. K. Laguaite, and J. W. Mclaurin, 'The hereditary syndrome of congenital deafness and retinitis pigmentosa (Usher's syndrome)', *The Laryngoscope*, 76:5 (1966), 850–62.

Kluchin, R. M., *Fit to be Tied: Sterilization and Reproductive Rights in America, 1950–1980* (New Brunswick, NJ: Rutgers University Press, 2011).

Kolb, L. C. and L. Roizin, *The First Psychiatric Institute: How Research and Education Changed Practice* (Washington, DC: American Psychiatric Press, Inc., 1993).

Konigsmark, B., *Hereditary Deafness in Man* (White Plains, NY: National Foundation, March of Dimes, 1969).

Krentz, C., *Writing Deafness: The Hearing Line in Nineteenth-century American Literature* (Chapel Hill, NC: University of North Carolina Press, 2007).

Ladd-Taylor, M., 'Eugenics, sterilisation and modern marriage in the USA: the strange career of Paul Popenoe', *Gender and History*, 13:2 (2001), 298–327.

Ladd-Taylor, M., '"A kind of genetic social work": Sheldon Reed and the origins of genetic counseling', in G. D. Feldberg (ed.), *Women, Health and Nation: Canada and the United States since 1945* (Montreal: McGill-Queen's University Press, 2003), pp. 67–83.

Lane, H., 'Cochlear implants: their cultural and historical meaning', in J. V. Van Cleve (ed.), *Deaf History Unveiled: Interpretations from the New Scholarship* (Washington, DC: Gallaudet University Press, 1993), pp. 273–91.

Lane, H., R. Hoffmeister, and B. J. Bahan, *A Journey into the Deaf-World* (San Diego, CA: DawnSignPress, 1996).

Lane, H. L., R. Pillard, and M. French, 'Origins of the American Deaf-world: Assimilating and differentiating societies and their relation to genetic patterning', *Sign Language Studies*, 1:1 (2000), 17–44.

Lane, H. L., R. Pillard, and U. Hedberg, *The People of the Eye: Deaf Ethnicity and Ancestry* (New York: Oxford University Press, 2011).

Levine, E., 'Historical review', in Rainer, Altshuler, and Kallmann (eds), *Family and Mental Health* (1963), pp. xvii–xxvi.

Lewontin, R. C., S. P. R. Rose, and L. J. Kamin, *Not in Our Genes: Biology, Ideology, and Human Nature* (New York: Pantheon Books, 1984).

Lindee, S. M., 'Genetic disease in the 1960s: a structural revolution, *American Journal of Medical Genetics*, 115:2 (2002), 75–82.

Lindee, S. M., *Moments of Truth in Genetic Medicine* (Baltimore, MD: Johns Hopkins University Press, 2005).

Linneaus, L., 'Heredity and intermarriage', *Volta Review*, 14 (1912), 184–6.

Lock, M. M. and V.-K. Nguyen, *An Anthropology of Biomedicine* (Chichester, West Sussex: Wiley-Blackwell, 2010).

Love, J. K., 'The study of the deaf child', *Volta Review*, 9 (1907), 449–64.

Loyd, J. M., *Health Rights Are Civil Rights: Peace and Justice Activism in Los Angeles, 1963–1978* (Minneapolis, MN: University of Minnesota Press, 2014).

Ludmerer, K. M., *Genetics and American Society: A Historical Appraisal.* (Baltimore, MD: Johns Hopkins University Press, 1972).

Lyons, S., 'College program leads way in deaf education. Western Maryland offers first Master's in sign language', *Baltimore Sun* (4 May 1998).

Maasen, S. and B. Sutter (eds), *On Willing Selves: Neoliberal Politics Vis-à-Vis the Neuroscientific Challenge* (Basingstoke: Palgrave Macmillan, 2007).

Mackenzie, C. D., *Alexander Graham Bell, the Man Who Contracted Space* (Boston, MA: Houghton Mifflin Company, 1928).

Macklin, M. T., 'Studies on the inheritance of deafness in the pupils of the Clarke School for the Deaf: genetic analysis of data and pedigrees', *The Laryngoscope*, 56:10 (1946), 583–601.

Marschark, M. and P. E. Spencer (eds), *Oxford Handbook of Deaf Studies, Language, and Education* (Oxford: Oxford University Press, 2003).

Mauldin, L., *Made to Hear: Cochlear Implants and Raising Deaf Children* (London: University of Minnesota Press, 2016).

McConnell, F., *The Bill Wilkerson Hearing and Speech Center, its Origin and its Development* (Nashville, TN: The Center, 1978).

McConnell, F. and Ward, P. H. (eds), *Deafness in Childhood* (Nashville, TN: Vanderbilt University Press, 1967).

McCulloch, J., *Black Soul, White Artifact: Fanon's Clinical Psychology and Social Theory* (Cambridge: Cambridge University Press, 1983).

Meckel, R. A., *Classrooms and Clinics: Urban Schools and the Protection and Promotion of Child Health, 1870-1930* (New Brunswick, NJ: Rutgers University Press, 2013).

Middleton, A., S. D. Emery, and G. H. Turner, 'Views, knowledge, and beliefs about genetics and genetic counseling among deaf people', *Sign Language Studies*, 10:2 (2010), 170-96.

Middleton, A., F. Robson, L. Burnell, and M. Ahmed, 'Providing a transcultural genetic counselling service in the UK', *Journal of Genetic Counseling*, 16:5 (2007), 567-82.

Miele Rodas, J., 'On blindness', *Journal of Cultural and Literary Disability Studies*, 3:2 (2009), 115-20.

Mildenberger, F., 'Auf der Spur des "scientific pursuit": Franz Josef Kallmann (1897-1965) und die rassenhygienische Forschung', *Medizinhistorisches Journal*, 37:2 (2002), 183-200.

Moeschen, S. C., 'Suffering silences, woeful afflictions: physical disability, melodrama, and the American Charity movement', *Comparative Drama*, 40:4 (2011), 433-54.

Murray, J., 'Genetics: a future peril facing the global deaf community', in H. Goodstein (ed.), *The Deaf Way II Reader: Perspectives from the Second International Conference on Deaf Culture* (Washington, DC: Gallaudet University Press, 2006), pp. 351-6.

Myklebust, H. R., *The Psychology of Deafness: Sensory Deprivation, Learning, and Adjustment* (New York: Grune & Stratton, 1964).

Nance, W. E., 'Genetic counseling for the hearing impaired', *Audiology: Official Organ of the International Society of Audiology*, 10:4 (1971), 222-33.

Nance, W. E., 'The principles and practice of genetic counseling', *The Annals of Otology, Rhinology, and Laryngology*, 80:2 (1971), 246-54.

Nance, W. E., 'Genetic aspects of Usher's syndrome', in *Symposium on Usher's Syndrome, D.C., April 19, 1973* (Washington, DC: Public Service Programs, Gallaudet College, 1973), pp. 12-18.

Nance, W. E., *What Every Person Should Know About Heredity and Deafness* (Washington, DC: Gallaudet College, 1975).

Nance, W. E., 'Studies of hereditary deafness', *Volta Review*, 78 (1976), 6-11.

Nance, W. E., 'Genetic counseling of hereditary deafness: an unmet need', in Bess (ed.), *Childhood Deafness* (1977), pp. 211-16.

Nance, W. E., 'The genetics of deafness', *Mental Retardation and Developmental Disabilities Research Reviews*, 9 (2003), 109-19.

Nance, W. E., 'The epidemiology of hereditary deafness: the impact of connexin 26 on the size and structure of the deaf community', in J. V. Van Cleve (ed.), *Genetics, Disability and Deafness* (Washington DC: Gallaudet University Press, 2004), pp. 94-105.

Nance, W. E. and M. J. Kearsey, 'Relevance of connexin deafness (DFNB1) to human evolution', *American Journal of Human Genetics*, 74:6 (2004), 1081-7.

Nance, W. E., J. B. Campbell, and F. R. Bieber, 'The Usher syndrome: a long neglected genetic disease', in Tully (ed.), *Workshop on Usher's Syndrome* (1977), pp. 4-7.

Nance, W. E., S. P. Rose, P. M. Conneally, and J. Z. Miller, 'Opportunities for genetic counseling through institutional ascertainment of affected probands', in H. A. Lubs and F. F. De la Cruz (eds), *Genetic Counseling* (New York: Raven Press: 1977), pp. 307–31.

National Institute on Deafness and Other Communication Disorders, 'Usher Syndrome', NIDCD Fact Sheet, www.nidcd.nih.gov/health/hearing/pages/usher. aspx#b [accessed 25 September 2018].

National Institutes of Health, *Proceedings: Conference on the Collection of Statistics of Severe Hearing Impairments and Deafness in the United States, 1964* (Washington, DC: U.S. Government Printing Office, 1964).

Nelson, A., *Body and Soul: The Black Panther Party and the Fight Against Medical Discrimination* (Minneapolis, MN: University of Minnesota Press, 2011).

Neugebauer, A., 'Hab ich das richtig verstanden. Den Möglichkeitsraum eingrenzen. Lippenlesen und Interaktion', in M. Schmidt and A. Werner (eds), *Zwischen Fremdbestimmung und Autonomie Neue Impulse zur Gehörlosengeschichte in Deutschland, Österreich und der Schweiz* (Bielefeld: Transcript, 2019), pp. 119–52.

Nielsen, K. E., *The Radical Lives of Helen Keller* (New York: New York University Press, 2009).

November, J. A., *Biomedical Computing: Digitizing Life in the United States* (Baltimore, MD: Johns Hopkins University Press, 2012).

Numbers, M. E., *My Words Fell on Deaf Ears: An Account of the First Hundred Years of the Clarke School for the Deaf* (Washington, DC: Alexander Graham Bell Association for the Deaf, 1974).

Numbers, R. L., *The Creationists* (New York: A. A. Knopf, 1992).

Osgood, R. L., *The History of Special Education: A Struggle for Equality in American Public Schools* (Westport, CT: Praeger, 2008).

Osgood, R. L., 'Education in the name of "improvement": the influence of eugenic thought and practice in Indiana's public schools, 1900–1930', *Indiana Magazine of History*, 106:3 (2010), 272–99.

Padden, C. A., 'Talking culture: Deaf people and Disability Studies', *Publications of the Modern Language Association of America*, 120:2 (2005), 508–13.

Padden, C. and T. Humphries, *Inside Deaf Culture* (Cambridge, MA: Harvard University Press, 2005).

Parens, E. and A. Asch, *Prenatal Testing and Disability Rights* (Washington, DC: Georgetown University Press, 2000).

Patterson, L., 'Points of access: rehabilitation centers, summer camps, and student life in the making of disability activism, 1960–1973', *Journal of Social History*, 46:2 (2012), 473–99.

Paul, D. B., *Controlling Human Heredity: 1865 to the Present* (Atlantic Highlands, NJ: Humanities Press, 1995).

Paul, D. B. and J. P. Brosco, *The PKU Paradox: A Short History of a Genetic Disease* (Baltimore, MD: Johns Hopkins University Press, 2014).

Petrina, S., 'The medicalization of education: a historiographic synthesis', *History of Education Quarterly*, 46:4 (2007), 503-31.
Pimentel, A., 'Handling the upper secondary and college Usher's syndrome student', in Tully (ed.), *Workshop on Usher's Syndrome* (1977), pp. 51-6.
Plotkin, S. A., 'The history of rubella and rubella vaccination leading to elimination', *Clinical Infectious Diseases: An Official Publication of the Infectious Diseases Society of America*, 43 (2005), 164-8.
Pols, H., 'War neurosis, adjustment problems in veterans, and an ill nation: the disciplinary project of American psychiatry during and after World War II', in G. Eghigian, A. Killen, and C. Leuenberger (eds), *The Self as Project: Politics and the Human Sciences* (Chicago, IL: University of Chicago Press, 2007), pp. 72-92.
Quaid, K. A., 'A few words from a "wise" woman', in Weir, Lawrence, and Fales (eds), *Genes and Human Self-knowledge* (1994), pp. 2-17.
Rainer, J. D., 'The contributions of Franz Josef Kallmann to the genetics of schizophrenia', *Behavioral Science*, 11:6 (1955), 413-37.
Rainer, J. D., 'Introduction', in Rainer, Altshuler, and Kallmann (eds), *Family and Mental Health* (1963), p. xiii.
Rainer, J. D., 'Background and history of New York State mental health program for the deaf', in Rainer and Altshuler (eds), *Psychiatry and the Deaf* (1968), pp. 1-4.
Rainer, J. D. and K. Z. Altshuler (eds), *Psychiatry and the Deaf: Workshop for Psychiatrists on Extending Mental Health Services to the Deaf* (Washington, DC: U.S. Department of Health, Education, and Welfare, Social and Rehabilitation Service, 1968).
Rainer, J. D. and K. Z. Altshuler, *Expanded Mental Health Care for the Deaf: Rehabilitation and Prevention* (Washington, DC: U.S. Department of Health, Education, and Welfare, Rehabilitation Services Administration, 1971).
Rainer, J. D. and W. E. Deming, 'Demographic aspects: number, distribution, marriage and fertility statistics', in Rainer, Altshuler, and Kallmann (eds), *Family and Mental Health* (1963), pp. 13-27.
Rainer, J. D. and F. J. Kallmann, 'Preventive mental health planning', in Rainer, Altshuler, and Kallmann (eds), *Family and Mental Health* (1963), pp. 217-27.
Rainer, J. D., K. Z. Altshuler, and F. J. Kallmann (eds), *Family and Mental Health Problems in a Deaf Population* (New York: New York State Psychiatric Unit, 1963).
Ramsden, E., 'Stress in the city: mental health, urban planning, and the social sciences in the post-war United States', in D. Cantor (ed.), *Stress, Shock, and Adaptation in the Twentieth Century* (Rochester, NY: University of Rochester Press, 2014), pp. 291-319.
Raz, A. E., *Community Genetics and Genetic Alliances: Eugenics, Carrier Testing and Networks of Risk* (London: Routledge, 2010).
Raz, M., 'Was cultural deprivation in fact sensory deprivation? Deprivation, retardation and intervention in the USA', *History of the Human Sciences*, 24:1 (2011), 51-69.
Raz, M., 'The deprivation riots: psychiatry as politics in the 1960s', *Harvard Review of Psychiatry*, 21:6 (2013), 345-50.

Reagan, L. J., *Dangerous Pregnancies: Mothers, Disabilities, and Abortion in America* (Berkeley, CA: University of California Press, 2010).

Reese, W. J., *Power and the Promise of School Reform: Grassroots Movements during the Progressive Era* (Boston, MA: Routledge & Kegan Paul, 1986).

Reilly, P., *The Surgical Solution: A History of Involuntary Sterilization in the United States* (Baltimore, MD: Johns Hopkins University Press, 1991).

Rembis, M., C. Kudlick, and K. E. Nielsen, 'Introduction', in M. Rembis, C. Kudlick, and K. E. Nielsen (eds), *The Oxford Handbook of Disability History* (New York: Oxford University Press, 2018), pp. 1–18.

Resta, R., 'The historical perspective: Sheldon Reed and 50 years of genetic counseling', *Journal of Genetic Counseling*, 6:4 (1996), 375–7.

Richardson, T. R., *The Century of the Child: The Mental Hygiene Movement and Social Policy in the United States and Canada* (Albany, NY: State University of New York Press, 1989).

Robinson, O., '"We are a different class": ableist rhetoric in deaf America 1880–1920', in S. Burch and A. Kafer (eds), *Deaf and Disability Studies: Interdisciplinary Perspectives* (Washington, DC: Gallaudet University Press, 2010), pp. 5–21.

Rocheleau, C. and R. Mack, *Those in Dark Silence: The Deaf-Blind in North America; a Record of To-Day* (Washington, DC: The Volta Bureau, 1930).

Roehrig, A., 'Coping with the discovery of Usher's syndrome' in *Symposium on Usher's Syndrome, D.C., April 19, 1973* (Washington, DC: Public Service Programs, Gallaudet College, 1973), pp. 32–8.

Roehrig, A., 'Living with Usher's syndrome', in Tully (ed.), *Workshop on Usher's Syndrome* (1977), pp. 23–7.

Roelcke, V., 'Die Etablierung der psychiatrischen Genetik in Deutschland, Grossbritannien und den USA, ca. 1910-1960: zur untrennbaren Geschichte von Eugenik und Humangenetik', *Vorträge und Abhandlungen Zur Wissenschaftsgeschichte* (2002/2003 and 2003/2004), 173–90.

Roelcke, V., 'Eugenic concerns, scientific practices: international relations and national adaptations in the establishment of psychiatric genetics in Germany, Britain, the USA, and Scandinavia 1910–1960', in B. M. Felder and P. Weindling (eds), *Baltic Eugenics: Bio-Politics, Race and Nation in Interwar Estonia, Latvia and Lithuania 1918–1940* (Amsterdam: Rodopi, 2013), pp. 301–33.

Roll-Hansen, N., 'The progress of eugenics: growth of knowledge and change in ideology', *History of Science*, 26 (1988), 295–331.

Rose, N. S., *Governing the Soul: The Shaping of the Private Self* (London: Routledge, 1990).

Rose, S. P., 'Genetic studies of profound prelingual deafness' (PhD dissertation, Indiana University, 1975).

Sank, D., 'Genetic aspects of early total deafness', in Rainer, Altshuler, and Kallmann (eds), *Family and Mental Health* (1963), pp. 28–81.

Schein, J. D., *The Deaf Community: Studies in the Social Psychology of Deafness* (Washington DC: Gallaudet College Press, 1968).

Schein, J. D., 'A brief history of services for deafblind people in the US', in C. L. Graham (ed.), *Transition Planning for Students Who Are DeafBlind* (Knoxville, TN: PEPNet-South, 2007), pp. 7–19.

Schlesinger, H., 'Cultural and environmental influences in the emotional development of the deaf', in Rainer and Altshuler (eds), *Psychiatry and the Deaf* (1968), pp. 128–31.

Schlesinger, L., 'The methods controversy in American deaf education: a sociological perspective' (Honor thesis, Smith College, 1977).

Schmidt, M. A., 'Extremely concerned and puzzled: hereditary deafness research at the Clarke School for the Deaf, 1930–1983', in B. H. Greenwald and J. J. Murray (eds), *In Our Own Hands: Essays in Deaf History, 1780–1970* (Washington, DC: Gallaudet University Press, 2016), pp. 193–209.

Schmidt, M. A., 'Planes of phenomenological experience: the psychology of deafness as an early example of American Gestalt psychology, 1928–1940', *History of Psychology*, 20:4 (2017), 347–64.

Schmidt, M. A., 'Birth defects, family dynamics, and mourning loss: psychoanalysis, genetic counseling and disability, 1950–1980', *Psychoanalysis and History*, 21:2 (2019), 147–69.

Schmidt, M. and A. Werner (eds), *Zwischen Fremdbestimmung und Autonomie Neue Impulse zur Gehörlosengeschichte in Deutschland, Österreich und der Schweiz* (Bielefeld: Transcript, 2019).

Schoeberlein, R. W., '"Maryland's shame": photojournalism and mental health reform, 1935–1949', *Maryland Historical Magazine*, 98:1 (2003), 34–72.

Schoen, J., *Choice & Coercion: Birth Control, Sterilization, and Abortion in Public Health and Welfare* (Chapel Hill, NC: University of North Carolina Press, 2005).

Schowe, B. M., 'Some observations on sign language', *Educational Research Bulletin*, 37:5 (1958), 120–4.

Schramm, K., D. Skinner, and R. Rottenburg (eds), *Identity Politics and the New Genetics: Re/creating Categories of Difference and Belonging* (New York: Berghahn Books, 2012).

Shambaugh, G. E., 'Discussion: medical treatment and research', in F. McConnell and P. H. Ward (eds), *Deafness in Childhood* (Nashville, TN: Vanderbilt University Press, 1967), pp. 252–62.

Shaver, K. A., J. A. Boughman, and W. E. Nance, 'LA antigens in the congenital Rubella syndrome', *Disease Markers*, 2 (1984), 381–91.

Shaver, K. A., J. A. Boughman, and W. E. Nance, 'Congenital rubella syndrome and diabetes: a review of epidemiologic, genetic, and immunologic factors', *American Annals of the Deaf*, 130:6 (1985), 526–32.

Shearer, A. E., M. S. Hildebrand, and R. J. H. Smith, 'Deafness and hereditary hearing loss overview', *NCBI Gene Reviews*, 1999, updated 27 July 2017, www.ncbi.nlm.nih.gov/books/NBK1434 [accessed 30 August 2018].

Shuttleworth, S., *The Mind of the Child: Child Development in Literature, Science, and Medicine, 1840–1900* (Oxford: Oxford University Press, 2010).

Silberman, S., *NeuroTribes: The Legacy of Autism and the Future of Neurodiversity* (New York: Avery, 2016).
Singer, J., *Neurodiversity: The Birth of an Idea* (Lexington, KY: n.p., 2017).
Sledzik, P. S., 'The Morris Steggerda Human Biology Collection', *National Museum of Health and Medicine, Armed Forces Institute of Pathology, Washington, DC, USA, Ethnographical Series*, 20 (2001), 281–6.
Small, J. G. and G. M. Desmarais, 'The familial occurrence of retinitis pigmentosa, mental disorders and EEG abnormalities', *The American Journal of Psychiatry*, 122:11 (1966), 1286–9.
Smith, D. J. and M. L. Wehmeyer, 'Who was Deborah Kallikak?', *Intellectual and Developmental Disabilities*, 50:2 (2012), 169–78.
Steggerda, M., R. Guilder, and L. A. Hopkins, *Report of the Research Department Concerning Heredity of Deafness* (Northampton, MA: Clarke School for the Deaf, 1931).
Stephens, S. D., 'Audiometers from Hughes to modern times', *British Journal of Audiology, Supplement*, 2 (1979), 17–23.
Stern, A. M., *Eugenic Nation: Faults and Frontiers of Better Breeding in Modern America* (Berkeley, CA: University of California Press, 2005).
Stern, A. M., *Telling Genes: The Story of Genetic Counseling in America* (Baltimore, MD: Johns Hopkins University Press, 2012).
Stokoe, W. C., *Sign Language Structure: An Outline of the Visual Communication Systems of the American Deaf* (Buffalo, NY: Department of Anthropology and Linguistics, University of Buffalo, 1960).
Stuckless, E. R., 'Rubella and the human burden', in E. M. Gruenberg, C. Lewis, and S. E. Goldston (eds), *Vaccinating Against Brain Syndromes: The Campaign Against Measles and Rubella* (New York: Oxford University Press, 1986), pp. 70–9.
Sussman, A. E. and L. G. Stewart, *Counseling with Deaf People* (New York: Deafness Research and Training Center, New York University School of Education, [1971] 1988).
Talaat, A., 'The Linda Annala, '70, scholarship', *Gallaudet University News*, 3 April 2017, www.gallaudet.edu/news/linda-annala-scholarship-fund [accessed 7 October 2018].
Taneja, P. R., A. Pandya, D. L. Foley, L. V. Niceley, and K. S. Arnos, 'Attitudes of deaf individuals towards genetic testing', *American Journal of Medical Genetics Part A*, 130A:1 (2004), 17–21.
Teslow, T., *Constructing Race: The Science of Bodies and Cultures in American Anthropology* (New York: Cambridge University Press, 2014).
Thomkins, A. V., 'Williams, Boyce R (1910–1998), advocate for deaf people, federal government official', in S. Burch, *Encyclopedia of American Disability History: Vol. 3* (New York: Facts On File, 2009), pp. 969–70.
Tinkle, W. J., 'Deafness as a eugenical problem' (doctoral dissertation, Ohio State University, 1932).
Tinkle, W. J., 'Deafness as a eugenic problem', *Journal of Heredity*, 24 (1933), 13–18.

Tomes, N., 'From outsiders to insiders: the consumer-survivor movement and its impact on U.S. mental health policy', in B. Hoffman, N. Tomes, R. Grob, and M. Schlesinger (eds), *Patients as Policy Actors* (New Brunswick, NJ: Rutgers University Press, 2011), pp. 112–31.

Torrie, C., 'Families with adolescent children with Usher's Syndrome: developing services to meet their needs', *American Annals of the Deaf*, special edition, 'Usher's syndrome: the personal, social, and emotional implication', ed. J. English, 123:3 (1978), 359–420.

Tuchman, A. M., 'Diabetes and "defective" genes in the twentieth-century United States', *Journal of the History of Medicine and Allied Sciences*, 70:1 (2013), 1–33.

Tucker, R., 'Coolidge Deaf Fund launched: school where Grace Goodhue taught is beneficiary', *Pittsburgh Press* (16 November 1928).

Tully, N. L. (ed.), *Papers Presented at Workshop on Usher's Syndrome, December 2–3, 1976. Conducted by Helen Keller National Center for Deaf-Blind Youths and Adults* (Sands Point, NY: Helen Keller National Center, 1977).

Usher, C. H., 'On the inheritance of retinitis pigmentosa, with notes of cases', *Royal London Ophthalmic Hospital Reports*, 19 (1914), 122–236.

Van Cleve, J. V. (ed.), *Genetics, Disability, and Deafness* (Washington, DC: Gallaudet University Press, 2004).

Van Cleve, J. V. and B. A. Crouch, *A Place of Their Own: Creating the Deaf Community in America* (Washington, DC: Gallaudet University Press, 1989).

Vernon, M., *Multiply Handicapped Deaf Children: Medical, Educational, and Psychological Considerations* (Washington, DC: Council for Exceptional Children, 1969).

Vernon, M., 'Usher's syndrome – deafness and progressive blindness: clinical cases, prevention, theory and literature survey', *Journal of Chronic Diseases*, 22:3 (1969), 133–51.

Vernon, M., 'The final report', in Grinker, *Psychiatric Diagnosis* (1971), pp. 13–37.

Vernon, M., 'Overview of Usher's syndrome: congenital deafness and progressive loss of vision', *Volta Review*, 76:2 (1974), 100–5.

Vernon, M., 'Usher's syndrome: problems and some solutions', *Hearing and Speech Action*, 44:4 (1976), 6–7, 9–13.

Vernon, M. and W. Hicks, 'A group counseling and educational program for students with Usher's syndrome', *Journal of Visual Impairment and Blindness*, 77:2 (1983), 64–6.

Vernon, M. and B. Makowsky, 'Deafness and minority group dynamics: sociological and psychological factors associated with hearing loss', *The Deaf American*, 21:11 (1969), 3–6.

Vernon, M., J. A. Boughman, and L. Annala, 'Considerations in diagnosing Usher's syndrome: RP and hearing loss', *Journal of Visual Impairment and Blindness*, 76:7 (1982), 258–61.

Vernon, M., L. E. Griswold, and Gallaudet College, *Usher's Syndrome: Retinitis Pigmentosa and Deafness* (Washington, DC: Gallaudet College, 1978).

Vidal, F. and F. Ortega, *Being Brains: Making the Cerebral Subject* (New York: Fordham University Press, 2017).

Volscho, T. W., 'Sterilization racism and pan-ethnic disparities of the past decade: the continued encroachment on reproductive rights', *Wicazo Sa Review*, 25:1 (2010), 17–31.

Waardenburg, P. J., 'A new syndrome combining developmental anomalies of the eyelids, eyebrows and nose root with pigmentary defects of the iris and head hair and with congenital deafness', *American Journal of Human Genetics*, 3:3 (1951), 195–253.

Wailoo, K., *Dying in the City of the Blues: Sickle Cell Anemia and the Politics of Race and Health* (Chapel Hill, NC: University of North Carolina Press, 2001).

Wailoo, K. and S. G. Pemberton, *The Troubled Dream of Genetic Medicine: Ethnicity and Innovation in Tay-Sachs, Cystic Fibrosis, and Sickle Cell Disease* (Baltimore, MD: Johns Hopkins University Press, 2006).

Weddle, B., *Mental Health in New York State, 1945–1998: A Historical Overview* (Albany, NY: The Archives, 2000).

Weir, R. F., S. C. Lawrence, and E. Fales (eds), *Genes and Human Self-Knowledge: Historical and Philosophical Reflections on Modern Genetics* (Iowa City: University of Iowa Press, 1994).

Werner, A., '"Double whammy"?! Historical glimpses of Black Deaf Americans', *COPAS*, 18:2 (2017), https://copas.uni-regensburg.de/article/view/288 [accessed 10 October 2019].

Wexler, A., *Mapping Fate: A Memoir of Family, Risk, and Genetic Research* (New York: Times Books, 1995).

Wildervanck, L. S., 'Hereditary malformations of the ear in three generations: marginal pits, pre-auricular appendages, malformations of the auricle and conductive deafness', *Acta Oto-Laryngologica*, 54 (1962), 1–6.

Wildervanck, L. S., 'The significance of associated anomalies in deafness, in *Reports of the Proceedings of the International Congress of the Deaf and the Forty-First Meeting of the Convention of American Instructors of the Deaf, Gallaudet College, Washington D.C. June 22–28 1963* (Washington, DC: U.S. Government Printing Office, 1964), pp. 632–8.

Williams, B., 'Salutatory statement', in J. D. Rainer (ed.), *Mental Health Planning for the Deaf, Report of a Conference of New York State Organizations for the Deaf, held at the New York State Psychiatric Institute on June 14, 1958* (New York, 1958), p. 205.

Wolfe, A. J., *Competing with the Soviets: Science, Technology, and the State in Cold War America* (Baltimore, MD: Johns Hopkins University Press, 2013).

Wortis, S. B. and D. Shaskan, 'Retinitis Pigmentosa and associated neuropsychiatric changes', *The Journal of Nervous and Mental Disease*, 92:4 (1940), 1990–1.

Wu, E. D., *Color of Success – Asian Americans and the Origins of the Model Minority* (Princeton, NJ: Princeton University Press, 2015).

Yale, C. A., *Years of Building: Memories of a Pioneer in a Special Field of Education* (New York: L. MacVeagh, The Dial Press, 1931).

Zames Fleischer, D. and F. Zames, *The Disability Rights Movement: From Charity to Confrontation* (Philadelphia, PA: Temple University Press, 2011).

Zamora, J. H., 'Hilde Schlesinger – UCSF Doctor, Deaf Advocate', *SF Gate* (October 7 2003).

Zenderland, A., *Measuring Minds: Henry Herbert Goddard and the Origins of American Intelligence Testing* (Cambridge: Cambridge University Press, 1998).

Zola, I. K., 'Helping one another: a speculative history of the self-help movement', *Archives of Physical Medicine and Rehabilitation*, 60:10 (1979), 452–6.

Zola, I. K., *Missing Pieces: A Chronicle of Living with a Disability* (Philadelphia, PA: Temple University Press, 1982).

Index

ableism 6, 11, 25, 36, 71, 95, 107–8, 114, 125, 170
activism 7, 11, 73, 84, 96, 100, 107–8, 110, 127–32, 139, 142–3, 176
Altshuler, Kenneth Z. 80, 90–2, 94, 98
American Society of Human Genetics 3, 51, 75
Annala, Linda 119, 122–4, 126–7
Arnos, Kathleen Shaver 12, 139, 148–60
audiology 5, 10, 36, 47–50, 54, 141–2
autonomy 24, 43, 98, 108–10, 121, 138, 144, 176

Bell, Alexander Graham 1–2, 21, 45, 49
   Clarke School for the Deaf 21, 29
   eugenics 5, 21–3
   Memoir Upon the Formation of a Deaf Variety of the Human Race 1–2, 21–2
   oralism 5, 21–2, 31
Best, Harry 27, 45
Bill Wilkerson Hearing and Speech Center (Nashville) 141–2
biomedical computing 59–60
Boughman, Joann A. 12, 119, 139, 143–53, 155–6, 160, 171
Brown, Kenneth 57–62, 65

chance 147–8, 157
   see also risk
Chung, Chin Sik 60–1
Clarence W. Barron research department 32–7
cochlear implants 166
connexin 26 deafness 1–2
Coolidge, Calvin 17, 29–30
Coolidge Fund for the Deaf 29–32, 47–50
Coolidge, Grace Goodhue 17, 29–30

Davenport, Charles 23, 47–8
Deaf ethnicity 174–5
   see also minority
deprivation research 87–90

empowerment 12, 125, 132, 139, 157–8, 161, 176
eugenics 6, 23–7, 47–8, 54, 71–2, 74–6
   deafness and 1, 5, 9–10, 17–18, 23, 25–7, 36, 43–44, 48–49, 51, 54–6, 64, 95, 98, 114, 118, 161, 169, 172–3, 176
Eugenics Record Office 10, 23, 47–50

Fay, Edgar Allen 45, 142
field work 150–1
   eugenic field workers 48–9
Friedman, Max 83–4, 91–2

Gallaudet University 108, 112, 121–3, 125, 127, 142–3, 149, 152
   Genetic Services Center 12, 153–61, 171–3
   Office of Demographic Studies 142–3
genetic counselling 7–8, 11–12, 43–44, 55–6, 62–4, 72, 93–98, 115, 118, 120–1, 131, 139–45, 156–61, 169–73, 179
   Clarke School for the Deaf 53–7, 64–5
   in sign language 139, 145–8, 152–56
genetic essentialism 175–6
genetic screening 65, 109, 115–18, 131, 155
Grinker, Roy 112–13
Guilder, Ruth Pierce 48–52, 54

Heider, Fritz, and Grace Moore Heider 10, 33–5, 37, 57, 78, 85–6, 168–9
Helen Keller Center 116, 123
heredity clinics 55–6
   see also genetic counselling
Hopkins, Louise Alice 48–59
Hudgins, Clarence V. 33, 57–9
Hudgins, Ruth B. 57

intermarriage 1–5, 10, 21–22, 25, 31, 44–6, 51–5, 60–5, 94, 169

INDEX

Kallmann, Franz Josef 10, 71–6, 79–80, 85–6, 91, 93–100, 156
Koffka, Kurt 32–3, 63

Levine, Edna Simon 78–9, 81–2, 85, 89, 112, 146
Lewis, Nolan D. C. 75

Macklin, Madge T. 51–3, 58, 63
manualism 19
  see also sign language
Mental Health Association of the Deaf 83–4
minority 6–7, 24
  deaf people as 2, 4, 9–11, 35, 71–3, 76, 79, 81, 83–5, 88–9, 92, 96–7, 99–100, 108, 112–13, 139, 143, 154, 160–1, 167–74
Myklebust, Helmer 87

Nance, Walter E. 1–3, 11–12, 121, 125–6, 138–45, 148–9, 153–6, 158, 160, 166, 171, 176
National Association of the Deaf (NAD) 25–6, 32, 123
National Institutes of Health (NIH) 10, 58–62, 149
  National Institute of Dental Research (NIDR) 58–9
  National Institute of Neurological Disease and Blindness 59
neuropsychiatry 113–14
  Usher syndrome and 107, 110–15, 130

Office of Vocational Rehabilitation (OVR) 79
oralism 5, 9–10, 18–22, 26, 30–7, 56, 81, 90–1, 108, 139, 141

psychology 18, 27
  of deafness 32–5, 37, 56, 78, 81, 85–8, 94, 98, 100, 108–10, 112, 119–22, 133, 143, 148, 157

Rainer, John D. 80, 86, 91, 93–8, 117
retinitis pigmentosa 107–8, 110–11, 117, 144
  see also Usher Syndrome

risk 12, 51, 53, 55, 62, 75, 96, 100, 109–10, 115, 118, 122, 130–2, 138–9, 143–4, 146–7, 154–7, 171–5
Rockland State Hospital 72
Roehrig, Arthur 122–4, 126, 128–9, 132, 146
rubella 113, 116–17, 139
  1964–65 epidemic 116
  chronic rubella syndrome (CRS) 110, 116, 149–51, 154
Rüdin, Ernst 74–5

Schein, Jerome D. 142–3
Schlesinger, Hilde 81, 89–90, 112–13
sign language 1–5, 19–22, 31, 35, 64, 66, 78, 90–2, 108, 113, 127, 138–9, 143, 166–7, 170–1, 175
  in genetic counselling 138–9, 145–8, 151–5, 160
  in psychiatry 10, 71, 91–2
  see also manualism
Smith College, Northampton 32–3, 47–9, 57
social model of disability and deafness 2–4, 7–8, 98, 114, 139, 154, 167–70
  see also minority
Steggerda, Morris 33, 43, 47–51, 58, 63
sterilization 6, 23–5, 27, 55, 64, 97–8
Stokoe, William 90
stress 86–8, 95, 100, 131
Sussman, Allen 84
syndromic deafness 8, 59, 61–2, 65, 109–11, 130

Tinkle, William J. 46, 49

Usher syndrome 11–12, 61, 107–32, 139–145, 152, 154, 170–1
  see also syndromic deafness

Vernon, McCay 107–21, 125, 130–1, 148, 170, 176

Wild, Henry D. 32, 34
Wildervanck, L. S. 61–2
Williams, Boyce 78–9, 81–82, 84

EU authorised representative for GPSR:
Easy Access System Europe, Mustamäe tee 50,
10621 Tallinn, Estonia
gpsr.requests@easproject.com

www.ingramcontent.com/pod-product-compliance
Lightning Source LLC
Chambersburg PA
CBHW070354240426
43671CB00013BA/2502